ANTI-INFLAMMATORY COOKBOOK FOR BEGINNERS

Elevate Your Immune system with 1000 Tasty, Healthy and Easy recipes to Reduce Inflammation and also Restore Your Body. 60 days meal plan

VICTOR WREN

Copyright © 2023 by Victor Wren

TABLE OF CONTENTS

INTRODUCTION

Step into a world of robust health and vitality as we introduce you to our book, **"ANTI-INFLAMMATORY COOKBOOK FOR BEGINNERS."** In this opening, we'll lay the foundation for your exploration of the rich content within this all-encompassing manual.

1. THE SIGNIFICANCE OF ADOPTING AN ANTI-INFLAMMATORY DIETARY APPROACH

Embarking on the exploration of the importance of an anti-inflammatory diet holds fundamental value for those new to the pursuit of enhanced health and well-being. Let's delve into the compelling rationales that underscore the relevance of embracing an anti-inflammatory diet.

A. Safeguarding Long-Term Health:
➤ **Elucidation**: An anti-inflammatory diet transcends momentary dietary preferences; it establishes a lifestyle that safeguards enduring health.

➤ **Illustrative Instance:** Through the consistent integration of anti-inflammatory foods, individuals have the potential to diminish the risk of chronic diseases, fostering comprehensive well-being.

B. Alleviating Chronic Inflammation:

➤ **Significance:** Chronic inflammation serves as the focal point for various health concerns, and an anti-inflammatory diet stands as a potent instrument to alleviate this prolonged inflammatory state.

➤ **Exemplification**: Persistent inflammation is intricately linked to conditions like cardiovascular diseases, diabetes, and arthritis. An anti-inflammatory diet directly addresses the foundational cause.

C. Fostering Holistic Well-Being:

➤ **Pertinence**: Beyond physical health, an anti-inflammatory diet fosters holistic well-being that encompasses mental and emotional dimensions.

➢ **Exemplary Scenario**: The nourishment derived from anti-inflammatory foods contributes to elevated mood, heightened energy levels, and augmented cognitive function.

D. Empowering the Body's Defense Mechanisms:
➢ **Significance**: An anti-inflammatory diet empowers the innate defense mechanisms of the body, rendering it more resilient to external stressors.
➢ **Concrete Representation:** Antioxidant-rich foods within the anti-inflammatory diet fortify the immune system, augmenting its capacity to fend off infections and illnesses.

E. Tackling the Root Causes of Inflammation:
➢ **Significance**: In contrast to merely addressing symptoms, an anti-inflammatory diet confronts the underlying causes of inflammation, offering a holistic approach to health.
➢ **Exemplary Case**: Instead of relying solely on pharmaceutical interventions for symptom relief, individuals can proactively modify their diet to curtail inflammation at its origin.

F. Prevention and Management of Chronic Conditions:

> **Relevance**: Embracing an anti-inflammatory diet represents a proactive stride in averting the onset of chronic conditions and effectively managing existing health challenges.
> **Exemplification:** Individuals contending with conditions such as rheumatoid arthritis may witness relief from symptoms and improvements in joint health through adherence to an anti-inflammatory eating plan.

G. Augmentation of Quality of Life:

> **Significance**: An anti-inflammatory diet contributes to an elevated quality of life by championing overall health and mitigating the repercussions of inflammatory conditions.
> **Example in Practice:** Individuals may encounter heightened mobility, diminished pain, and a sense of vitality, positively influencing their day-to-day lives.

H. Empowerment Through Informed Choices:
> **Importance**: Grasping the significance of an anti-inflammatory diet empowers individuals to make discerning choices regarding their dietary habits.
> **Concretized Understanding:** Armed with insights into the impact of diverse foods on inflammation, individuals can make conscious decisions that align with their health objectives.

In essence, the adoption of an anti-inflammatory diet matters because it transcends transient trends and short-term solutions. It lays the groundwork for enduring health, resilience, and an overall enriched quality of life. For beginners, this comprehension serves as a portal to a journey of mindful eating and holistic well-being.

2. EXPLORING THE BENEFITS OF EMBRACING AN ANTI-INFLAMMATORY DIET

Embarking on the path of an anti-inflammatory diet provides a myriad of advantages that go beyond merely diminishing inflammation. Delving into these advantages is crucial for novices who seek to grasp the affirmative influence this dietary strategy can exert on overall health and well-being.

A. Inflammation Minimization for Enhanced Health:

> **Importance**: The primary objective of an anti-inflammatory diet is to decrease persistent inflammation.
> **Example**: Augmented intake of fruits and vegetables, teeming with antioxidants, aids in pacifying inflammation within the body.

B. Enhancement of Cardiovascular Health:

> **Positive Impact:** Embracing an anti-inflammatory diet actively contributes to the well-being of the heart.
> **Illustration**: Omega-3 fatty acids derived from sources like fatty fish are correlated with diminished risks of heart ailments.

C. Maintenance of Balanced Blood Sugar Levels:

> **Effect**: An anti-inflammatory diet assists in maintaining stable blood sugar levels.
> **Example**: Consumption of whole grains and foods rich in fiber prevents abrupt spikes and declines in blood glucose.

D. Promotion of Joint Health:

➤ **Advantage:** Anti-inflammatory foods exert a positive influence on conditions affecting the joints.

➤ **Illustrative Scenario:** The inclusion of turmeric, acknowledged for its anti-inflammatory attributes, may alleviate symptoms in individuals grappling with arthritis.

E. Support for Weight Management:

➤ **Effectiveness**: An anti-inflammatory diet actively contributes to the regulation of weight.

➤ **Exemplar**: Prioritizing whole foods and incorporating lean proteins fosters a feeling of fullness, facilitating weight maintenance.

F. Boosting Cognitive Function:

➤ **Positive Influence**: Foods with anti-inflammatory properties may contribute to cognitive well-being.

➤ **Example**: Diets abundant in nutrients like omega-3 fatty acids, known for their brain-boosting potential, are associated with improved cognitive function.

G. Fostering Digestive System Well-Being:
- ➤ **Advocacy**: An anti-inflammatory diet advocates for the well-being of the digestive system.
- ➤ **Illustration**: Integration of probiotic-rich foods aids in preserving a diverse and beneficial gut microbiome.

H. Heightened Energy Levels:
- ➤ **Effect**: Providing the body with anti-inflammatory foods amplifies overall energy.
- ➤ **Example**: Well-balanced meals incorporating a variety of nutrients ensure sustained energy throughout the day.

I. Reinforcement of Immune Function:
- ➤ **Fortification**: Anti-inflammatory foods positively fortify the immune system.
- ➤ **Exemplification**: Essential vitamins and antioxidants present in fruits and vegetables contribute significantly to immune support.

J. Cultivation of Overall Well-Being:
- ➤ **Holistic Influence:** Embracing an anti-inflammatory diet nurtures a profound sense of vitality.
- ➤ **Illustrative Outcome:** Individuals frequently express heightened energy levels, enhanced focus, and emotional equilibrium when adhering to an anti-inflammatory dietary regimen.

Exploring the advantages of an anti-inflammatory diet not only illuminates its potential in countering inflammation but also underscores its comprehensive influence on diverse facets of health. For beginners, this comprehension serves as inspiration to adopt a dietary methodology that not only pleases the palate but also contributes to enduring well-being.

3. A GUIDE ON HOW TO MAKE THE MOST OF THIS COOKBOOK

This cookbook goes beyond being a mere compilation of recipes; it serves as your detailed guide to achieving improved well-being. We'll furnish you with precise guidance on how to maximize the use of this cookbook, helping you smoothly navigate its diverse sections and leverage it as a powerful tool for your journey towards better health. Whether you boast culinary expertise or are a newcomer to the kitchen, this guide is customized to meet your specific needs.

4. DELVING DEEPER INTO THE IMPACT OF INFLAMMATION ON YOUR HEALTH

Before embarking on our culinary adventure, it's crucial to grasp the underlying causes of inflammation and its significant impact on your overall health. We'll closely examine what inflammation is, its associations with various health conditions, and the compelling reasons why you should aim to reduce it through your dietary and lifestyle choices.

Armed with these foundational insights, you're well-prepared to journey through the subsequent chapters. From comprehending the science of anti-inflammatory nutrition to crafting a comprehensive 60-day meal plan, exploring exercise regimens, and honing your skills in anti-inflammatory cooking techniques, this book empowers you with the knowledge and expertise essential to embrace a healthier, inflammation-free life.

So, let's embark on this exciting and transformative path to enhanced well-being as you explore the pages of **"ANTI-INFLAMMATORY COOKBOOK FOR BEGINNERS."** Your journey to a healthier, more vibrant you begins now.

CHAPTER 1
UNDERSTANDING THE ANTI-INFLAMMATORY DIET

1.1. WHAT IS INFLAMMATION AND ITS ROLE IN HEALTH?

Inflammation constitutes an inherent and indispensable aspect of the body's defense apparatus. It embodies the immune system's reaction to injury, infection, or detrimental stimuli. Whereas immediate inflammation is a safeguarding and localized retort directed at eradicating the root cause of cellular injury, persistent inflammation, conversely, may exert adverse effects on health.

A. Immediate Inflammation:
- ➢ **Description**: An expeditious and ephemeral reaction to injuries or infections.
- ➢ **Objective**: Mobilizes immune cells, blood vessels, and molecular mediators to the impacted region for a precise defense.
- ➢ **Illustrations**: Swelling and redness following a laceration, the sensation of warmth encircling an injury.

B. Prolonged Inflammation:

➤ **Definition**: An extended and continual inflammatory response enduring for weeks, months, or even years.

➤ **Triggers**: Persistent infections, autoimmune disorders, protracted exposure to irritants, and lifestyle factors such as suboptimal diet and stress.

➤ **Health Ramifications:** Persistent inflammation correlates with various health conditions, encompassing cardiovascular diseases, diabetes, arthritis, and specific cancers.

C. Function of Inflammation in Health:

i. Shielding Against Infections:

➤ Inflammation constitutes an integral component of the body's defense against deleterious pathogens.

➤ White blood cells are prompted to obliterate invading microorganisms.

ii. Reparation and Healing of Tissues:

➢ Following an injury, inflammation aids in purging damaged cells and instigating the recuperative process.

➢ It fosters the regeneration of novel, robust tissue.

iii. Activation of the Immune System:

➢ Inflammation triggers immune cells to identify and nullify threats.

➢ It assumes a role in the body's immune surveillance.

iv. Resolution of Infections:

➢ Inflammation assists in isolating and eradicating infectious agents.

➢ Once the threat is neutralized, the inflammatory response should ideally diminish.

D. Harmonizing Inflammation for Optimal Health:

➢ While inflammation serves as an imperative defense mechanism, persistent inflammation may precipitate health complications.

➢ Dietary and lifestyle choices wield substantial influence in either fostering or mitigating inflammation.

➢ The anti-inflammatory diet concentrates on assimilating foods that can assist in modulating the inflammatory response and fostering overall well-being.

Apprehending the dualistic nature of inflammation furnishes novices with the understanding to acknowledge its pivotal role in health while proactively averting chronic inflammation through conscientious lifestyle choices and dietary preferences.

Consider your body like a bustling city. Acute inflammation is like a brief, localized police response to a minor incident. Chronic inflammation, on the other hand, is an ongoing state of heightened alert, leading to stress on the city's resources and infrastructure.

1.2. THE SCIENCE BEHIND ANTI-INFLAMMATORY EATING

Delving into the scientific underpinnings of anti-inflammatory eating unveils the intricate mechanisms that dictate how certain foods influence inflammation levels in the body. This comprehension empowers beginners to make informed dietary choices conducive to reducing inflammation.

A. Inflammatory Pathways:

➤ **Explanation**: The body's inflammatory response involves complex signaling pathways.

➤ Illustration: Omega-3 fatty acids found in fatty fish (e.g., salmon) have been shown to modulate inflammation by inhibiting specific pro-inflammatory pathways.

B. Nutrient Influence on Inflammation:

➤ **Insight**: Various nutrients play pivotal roles in either promoting or mitigating inflammation.

- **Example**: Curcumin, present in turmeric, possesses anti-inflammatory properties, hindering the activity of inflammatory molecules.

C. Gut Microbiota and Inflammation:

➢ **Understanding**: The gut microbiota profoundly impacts inflammation levels in the body.

➢ **Instance**: Probiotics, found in yogurt, contribute to a healthy gut microbiome, potentially reducing inflammation.

D. Role of Antioxidants:

➢ **Clarification**: Antioxidants combat oxidative stress, a contributor to inflammation.

➢ **Case in Point**: Berries, rich in antioxidants like anthocyanins, are linked to lower levels of inflammatory markers.

E. Impact of Processed Foods:

➢ **Insight**: Highly processed foods may contribute to inflammation.

➢ **Exemplification**: Trans fats, prevalent in many processed snacks, have been associated with an increased inflammatory response.

F. Balancing Omega-6 and Omega-3 Fatty Acids:

➢ **Explanation**:Maintaining a balance between these fatty acids is crucial for inflammation control.

➢ **Example**: Nuts and seeds, while sources of omega-6, can be part of a balanced diet when paired with omega-3-rich foods like flaxseeds or fatty fish.

G. Inflammatory Foods and Conditions:

➢ **Association**: Certain foods are linked to inflammatory conditions.

➢ **Illustrative Link:** High consumption of refined sugars, as found in sugary beverages and desserts, has been correlated with increased inflammation and related health issues.

Understanding the scientific intricacies behind anti-inflammatory eating empowers individuals to make choices that positively influence inflammation levels in the body. By incorporating foods with anti-inflammatory properties, beginners embark on a journey toward improved well-being and overall health.

Think of antioxidants as the firefighters of your body. They rush to the scene of inflammation to put out the fire and ensure your cells remain unharmed.

1.3. CHRONIC INFLAMMATION AND ITS HEALTH IMPLICATIONS

Delving into the repercussions of persistent inflammation is indispensable for newcomers traversing the route to an anti-inflammatory way of life. Chronic inflammation, enduring over an elongated span, can markedly influence well-being and contribute to an array of conditions.

A. Definition of Chronic Inflammation:

➢ **Elucidation**: An extended and sustained inflammatory response persisting for weeks, months, or even years.

➢ **Importance**: Chronic inflammation deviates from the body's typical state, potentially resulting in adverse effects on health.

B. Origins of Chronic Inflammation:

➢ **Factors at Play**: Ongoing infections, autoimmune maladies, prolonged exposure to irritants, and lifestyle elements such as an insufficient diet and persistent stress.

➢ **Illustration**: Persistent contact with environmental pollutants could incite chronic inflammation.

C. Health Ramifications of Persistent Inflammation:

i. Cardiovascular Diseases:

➢ **Relation**: Chronic inflammation is associated with an elevated risk of heart maladies.

➢ **Depiction**: Increased levels of inflammatory markers may contribute to the initiation of atherosclerosis.

ii. Diabetes:

➢ **Connection**: Chronic inflammation might contribute to insulin resistance.

➢ Example: Inflammation within adipose tissue has been associated with the onset of type 2 diabetes.

iii. Arthritis:

➢ **Association**: Chronic inflammation is pivotal in the advancement of arthritis.

➢ **Instance**: Rheumatoid arthritis manifests as chronic inflammation affecting the joints.

iv. Certain Cancers:

➤ **Link**: Persistent inflammation might foster the commencement and progression of select cancers.

➤ **Representative Scenario:** Chronic inflammation within the gastrointestinal tract correlates with an augmented risk of colorectal cancer.

D. Neurological Implications:

➤ **Observation**: Persistent inflammation could hold consequences for neurological well-being.

➤ **Exemplary Case:** Research is exploring inflammatory processes in the brain concerning neurodegenerative conditions like Alzheimer's disease.

E. Impact on Mental Health:

➤ **Recognition**: Chronic inflammation is under examination for its conceivable role in mental health conditions.

➤ **Instance**: Studies propose a relationship between inflammation and disorders such as depression and Anxiety.

Comprehending the aftermath of chronic inflammation underscores the necessity of embracing an anti-inflammatory lifestyle. Through deliberate dietary selections and lifestyle adjustments, novices can proactively take measures to alleviate persistent inflammation, fostering enduring health and well-being.

Chronic inflammation is like the persistent drip from a leaky pipe in your home. Over time, it damages the foundation, and you end up with structural issues. Similarly, chronic inflammation damages your body's foundation, leading to various health concerns.

1.4. THE POSITIVE IMPACT OF AN ANTI-INFLAMMATORY DIET ON YOUR HEALTH

Exploring the affirmative outcomes of adopting an anti-inflammatory diet is pivotal for beginners on their journey toward improved well-being. The deliberate inclusion of anti-inflammatory foods can lead to a spectrum of positive impacts on various aspects of health.

A. Reduction in Inflammation Levels:

➤ **Observation**: An anti-inflammatory diet is designed to mitigate chronic inflammation.

➤ **Example**: Increased consumption of fatty fish rich in omega-3 fatty acids has been linked to lower levels of inflammatory markers.

B. Cardiovascular Health Improvement:

➤ **Effect**: Adopting an anti-inflammatory diet may contribute to heart health.

➤ **Illustration**: Diets rich in fruits, vegetables, and whole grains have been associated with a reduced risk of cardiovascular diseases.

C. Better Blood Sugar Control:

➤ **Impact**: An anti-inflammatory diet may assist in regulating blood sugar levels.

➤ **Example**: Consuming fiber-rich foods like legumes and whole grains can help stabilize blood glucose levels.

D. Joint Health Enhancement:

➤ **Outcome**: Anti-inflammatory foods can positively affect joint conditions.

➤ **Illustrative** Scenario: Increased intake of anti-inflammatory spices like turmeric has been linked to reduced symptoms in individuals with arthritis.

E. Weight Management Support:

➤ **Effectiveness**: An anti-inflammatory diet may aid in weight control.

➤ **Exemplar**: Incorporating lean proteins and whole foods can contribute to a balanced and satiating diet, supporting weight maintenance.

F. Brain Health Preservation:

➤ **Positive Influence:** Anti-inflammatory foods may play a role in cognitive well-being.

➤ **Example**: Diets rich in antioxidants, prevalent in berries and leafy greens, have been associated with cognitive benefits.

G. Gut Health Optimization:
> **Enhancement**: An anti-inflammatory diet promotes a healthy gut microbiome.
> **Illustration**: Probiotic-rich foods like yogurt can foster a diverse and beneficial gut microbial community.

H. Improved Energy Levels:
> **Effect**: Nourishing the body with anti-inflammatory foods may boost overall energy.
> **Example**: Whole grains and lean proteins provide sustained energy, avoiding energy spikes and crashes.

I. Enhanced Immune Function:
> **Strengthening**: Anti-inflammatory foods can positively influence immune responses.
> **Exemplification**: Vitamin C-rich foods, such as citrus fruits, contribute to immune system support.

J. Overall Well-Being and Vitality:

> ➤ **Holistic Impact**: Embracing an anti-inflammatory diet contributes to a sense of overall health and vitality.

> ➤ **Illustrative Outcome**: Individuals often report increased energy, improved mood, and a general sense of well-being after adopting an anti-inflammatory eating plan.

Knowing the myriad ways in which an anti-inflammatory diet can positively impact health serves as motivation for beginners to make sustainable dietary choices, fostering a journey towards lasting well-being and vitality.

Picture your body as a car. When supplied with the appropriate fuel, subjected to consistent upkeep, and equipped with a pristine engine, your body operates seamlessly and optimally. An anti-inflammatory diet serves as the premium-grade fuel and upkeep regimen essential for the efficient functioning your body requires.

1.5. EXPLORING THE CONNECTION BETWEEN YOUR MIND AND BODY:

STRESS AND INFLAMMATION

Delving into the intricate interplay between the mind and body unveils a significant connection between stress and inflammation. Recognizing this relationship is essential for beginners navigating the path toward an anti-inflammatory lifestyle.

A. Understanding the Stress-Inflammation Nexus:

> **Insight**: Stress, whether chronic or acute, can influence the body's inflammatory responses.
> **Example**: High-stress situations may trigger the release of stress hormones, contributing to an inflammatory reaction.

B. Impact of Chronic Stress on Inflammation:

> **Observation**: Prolonged or chronic stress may contribute to persistent inflammation.
> **Illustration**: Individuals experiencing chronic stressors, such as work-related pressures, may exhibit elevated inflammatory markers.

C. Psychological Stressors and Inflammatory Response:

> **Connection**: Psychological stressors, including anxiety and depression, can influence inflammation.
> **Example**: Studies suggest that individuals with chronic psychological stress may have increased inflammatory activity.

D. Stress-Induced Inflammatory Hormones:

> **Mechanism**: Stress activates the release of hormones that can trigger inflammation.
> **Illustrative Scenario**: Cortisol, the primary stress hormone, has been linked to increased inflammation when chronically elevated.

E. Mind-Body Practices to Reduce Inflammation:

> **Approach**: Mindfulness, meditation, and relaxation techniques can mitigate stress and potentially reduce inflammation.
> **Example**: Engaging in regular mindfulness meditation has shown to have anti-inflammatory effects.

F. Nutritional Impact on Stress and Inflammation:
- ➤ **Influence:** Dietary choices can either exacerbate or alleviate the impact of stress on inflammation.
- ➤ **Illustration**: Consuming a diet rich in anti-inflammatory foods may provide resilience against stress-induced inflammation.

G. Stress Management Strategies for an Anti-Inflammatory Lifestyle:
- ➤ **Recommendations**: Integrating stress management practices is crucial for an anti-inflammatory approach.
- ➤ **Example**: Incorporating activities like yoga or deep-breathing exercises into daily routines can contribute to stress reduction.

H. Holistic Well-Being:
- ➤ **Recognition**: Addressing both mental and physical aspects is key to overall well-being.
- ➤ **Illustrative Outcome**: Individuals practicing stress-reduction techniques while adopting an anti-inflammatory diet often report enhanced overall health and vitality.

Understanding the intricate connection between stress and inflammation empowers beginners to adopt a holistic approach to well-being. By implementing stress-management strategies alongside an anti-inflammatory diet, individuals can foster a harmonious balance between mind and body, promoting enduring health and resilience.

In this chapter, we've established the foundation for your venture into the realm of anti-inflammatory nutrition. You've gained insights into the dual nature of inflammation, understanding its role as both a protagonist and antagonist. We've explored how an anti-inflammatory diet can harness this power and the profound implications it holds for your well-being. Now, let's delve into the pragmatic facets of this journey – from dietary choices and avoidance strategies to exercises that actively mitigate inflammation and beyond. Your initiation into a healthier, inflammation-free life is just commencing.

CHAPTER 2
WHAT TO EAT AND WHAT TO AVOID

2.1. A COMPREHENSIVE FOOD LIST

Embracing an anti-inflammatory lifestyle involves making mindful choices about the foods you consume. This comprehensive food list will guide you in selecting ingredients that support your journey towards reducing inflammation. Consider it your guide for procuring elements that contribute to enhanced well-being. As you explore this array, you'll uncover a realm of ingredients that not only tantalize your taste buds but also bring the added advantage of diminishing inflammation within your body.

Picture a rainbow of fruits and vegetables – from vibrant red tomatoes to deep green kale, and golden turmeric.

These are your anti-inflammatory allies, each with unique benefits.

★ **Fruits**:

1. Berries:
    - Blueberries
    - Strawberries
    - Raspberries

2. Cherries

3. Citrus Fruits:
    - Oranges
    - Grapefruits
    - Lemons
    - Limes

4. Pineapple

5. Papaya

6. Avocado

7. Apples

8. Watermelon

9. Grapes

★ **Vegetables**:
1. Leafy Greens:
   - Spinach
   - Kale
   - Swiss Chard

2. Cruciferous Vegetables:
   - Broccoli
   - Cauliflower
   - Brussels Sprouts

3. Root Vegetables:
   - Sweet Potatoes
   - Carrots

4. Bell Peppers

5. Tomatoes

6. Cucumbers

7. Zucchini

8. Mushrooms

★ **Whole Grains**:

1. Quinoa

2. Brown Rice

3. Oats

4. Barley

5. Buckwheat

6. Whole Wheat

7. Farro

★ **Legumes**:

1. Lentils

2. Chickpeas

3. Black Beans

4. Kidney Beans

5. Pinto Beans

6. Edamame

★ Nuts and Seeds:

1. Almonds

2. Walnuts

3. Chia Seeds

4. Flaxseeds

5. Hemp Seeds

6. Sunflower Seeds

★ Fatty Fish:

1. Salmon

2. Mackerel

3. Sardines

4. Trout

5. Herring

★ Lean Proteins:

1. Skinless Poultry:
   - Chicken
   - Turkey

2. Lean Cuts of Beef or Pork

3. Tofu

4. Tempeh

★ Dairy and Dairy Alternatives:
1. Greek Yogurt

2. Kefir

3. Almond Milk

4. Coconut Milk (unsweetened)

★ Healthy Fats:
1. Extra Virgin Olive Oil

2. Avocado Oil

3. Flaxseed Oil

4. Coconut Oil

★ Herbs and Spices:
1. Turmeric

2. Ginger

3. Garlic

4. Cinnamon

5. Rosemary

6. Basil

7. Parsley

★ Beverages:

1. Green Tea

2. Herbal Teas:
   - Chamomile
   - Peppermint

3. Water with Lemon

Use this comprehensive food list as your culinary compass, exploring a variety of flavors and ingredients to create nourishing and anti-inflammatory meals.

2.2. DETAILED LIST OF ANTI-INFLAMMATORY FOODS

To harness the full potential of an anti-inflammatory diet, you need to know your allies intimately. We will furnish you with an intricate compilation of foods recognized for their anti-inflammatory properties, elucidating the scientific rationale behind the efficacy of each as a potent combatant against inflammation. Whether it's the omega-3 fatty acids abundant in fatty fish or the antioxidants present in blueberries, you'll gain a substantial reservoir of information to inform and steer your dietary preferences.

Example: Omega-3 fatty acids are like the knights in shining armor, defending your body against inflammation. They're found in salmon, walnuts, and flaxseeds, ready to protect your health.

This detailed list provides a comprehensive guide to anti-inflammatory foods, offering variety and flavor while promoting health.

★ FRUITS:

1. Berries:
    - Blueberries
    - Strawberries
    - Raspberries

2. Cherries

3. Citrus Fruits:
    - Oranges
    - Grapefruits
    - Lemons
    - Limes

4. Pineapple

5. Papaya

6. Avocado

7. Apples

8. Watermelon

9. Grapes

★ VEGETABLES

1. Leafy Greens:
   - Spinach
   - Kale
   - Swiss Chard

2. Cruciferous Vegetables:
   - Broccoli
   - Cauliflower
   - Brussels Sprouts

3. Root Vegetables:
   - Sweet Potatoes
   - Carrots

4. Bell Peppers

5. Tomatoes

6. Cucumbers

7. Zucchini

8. Mushrooms

★ WHOLE GRAINS:

1. Quinoa

2. Brown Rice

3. Oats

4. Barley

5. Buckwheat

6. Whole Wheat

7. Farro

★ LEGUMES:

1. Lentils

2. Chickpeas

3. Black Beans

4. Kidney Beans

5. Pinto Beans

6. Edamame

★ NUTS AND SEEDS:

1. Almonds

2. Walnuts

3. Chia Seeds

4. Flaxseeds

5. Hemp Seeds

6. Sunflower Seeds

★ FATTY FISH:

1. Salmon

2. Mackerel

3. Sardines

4. Trout

5. Herring

★ LEAN PROTEINS :

1. Skinless Poultry:
   - Chicken
   - Turkey

2. Lean Cuts of Beef or Pork

3. Tofu

4. Tempeh

★ DAIRY AND DAIRY ALTERNATIVES:

1. Greek Yogurt

2. Kefir

3. Almond Milk

4. Coconut Milk (unsweetened)

★ HEALTHY FATS:

1. Extra Virgin Olive Oil

2. Avocado Oil

3. Flaxseed Oil

4. Coconut Oil

★ HERBS AND SPICES:

1. Turmeric

2. Ginger

3. Garlic

4. Cinnamon

5. Rosemary

6. Basil

7. Parsley

★ BEVERAGES:

1. Green Tea

2. Herbal Teas:
    - Chamomile
    - Peppermint

3. Water with Lemon

This detailed list empowers beginners to navigate the world of anti-inflammatory foods, promoting a diverse and delicious approach to a healthier lifestyle. Explore these ingredients, experiment with flavors, and embrace the benefits of an anti-inflammatory diet.

2.3. FOODS TO LIMIT OR AVOID

In your journey toward an anti-inflammatory lifestyle, being mindful of certain foods can further support your health goals. Within this segment, we will delve into the realm of foods that have the potential to exacerbate inflammation. Frequently, these items are rich in sugar, detrimental fats, and synthetic additives. Through the recognition and restriction of these offenders, you'll edge closer to realizing your health objectives.

Example: Processed foods laden with trans fats and refined sugars are like the villains of your anti-inflammatory story. They sneak in, causing chaos and inflammation within your body.

Here's a guide to foods that are best enjoyed in moderation or avoided to promote overall well-being.

★ **PROCESSED FOODS**:

1. Highly Processed Snacks:
   - Chips
   - Crackers with additives
   - Packaged cookies

2. Sugary Cereals:
   - Those high in added sugars
   - Low-fiber options

3. Fast Food:
   - Burgers
   - Fries
   - Fried chicken

4. Processed Meats:
   - Sausages
   - Hot dogs
   - Bacon

★ REFINED CARBOHYDRATES:

1. White Bread:
   - Opt for whole grain alternatives.

2. White Rice:
   - Choose brown rice or other whole grains.

3. Pastries:
   - Doughnuts
   - Croissants
   - Sweet pastries

4. Sugary Beverages:
   - Soda
   - Sweetened fruit drinks
   - Energy drinks

SATURATED AND TRANS FATS:

1. Fried Foods:
   - French fries
   - Fried chicken
   - Fried snacks

2. Margarine:
   - High in trans fats

3. Shortening:
   - Often found in processed baked goods

4. Processed Baked Goods:
   - Commercial cakes
   - Cookies
   - Pastries

★ EXCESSIVE RED MEAT:

1. Red Meat:
   - Limit consumption, especially processed varieties.

★ SUGARY TREATS :

1. Candies:
   - High-sugar candies
   - Candy bars

2. Pastries:
   - Doughnuts
   - Sweet rolls

3. Sweetened Desserts:
   - Cakes
   - Pies
   - Ice cream with added sugars

★ EXCESSIVE DAIRY :

1. Full-Fat Dairy Products:
   - Whole milk
   - Full-fat cheeses
   - Cream

★ ARTIFICIAL ADDITIVES :

1. Artificial Sweeteners:
   - Saccharin, aspartame, sucralose

2. High-Fructose Corn Syrup:
   - Found in many processed foods

3. Artificial Colorings and Flavorings:
   - Check ingredient labels for additives

Being mindful of these foods will empower you to make choices that align with your anti-inflammatory goals. As you embark on your culinary journey, focus on incorporating nourishing and whole foods to support your overall health and well-being.

2.4. NAVIGATING FOOD LABELS:
MAKING INFORMED CHOICES

Understanding how to decipher food labels is crucial for making informed choices on your anti-inflammatory journey. This section provides a guide to reading labels, empowering you to select foods that align with your health goals.

Example: Ever seen a long list of unpronounceable ingredients on a label? It's like a puzzle waiting to be solved. We'll give you the tools to decode the puzzle and make the healthiest choices.

1. Check the Ingredients List:
- Prioritize foods with fewer and recognizable ingredients.
- Be cautious of long lists with additives and preservatives.

2. Mindful of Added Sugars:
- Look for alternative names for sugar (e.g., sucrose, high-fructose corn syrup).
- Opt for products with minimal added sugars.

3. Watch Out for Unhealthy Fats:
- Avoid trans fats and limit saturated fats.
- Choose products with healthier fats like monounsaturated and polyunsaturated fats.

4. Assess Sodium Content:
- High sodium intake may contribute to inflammation.
- Select products with lower sodium levels.

5. Understand Serving Sizes:
- Be aware of portion sizes to accurately assess nutritional content.
- Adjust values based on your serving size.

6. Look for Whole Grains:
- Choose products with whole grains as the first ingredient.
- Terms like "whole wheat" and "whole grain" indicate healthier options.

7. Check for Artificial Additives:
- Be wary of artificial colors, sweeteners, and preservatives.
- Opt for products with natural ingredients.

8. Consider Allergens:
- Identify potential allergens if applicable.
- Ensure the product aligns with your dietary needs.

9. Evaluate Nutrient Content:
- Focus on products rich in essential nutrients (vitamins, minerals, fiber).
- Ensure nutritional content supports your dietary requirements.

10. Be Skeptical of Health Claims:
- Question products with exaggerated health claims.
- Rely on the ingredient list and nutritional information for accuracy.

11. Choose Local and Organic Options:
- Local and organic products may have fewer additives.
- Support sustainable and environmentally friendly choices.

Navigating food labels empowers you to make conscious choices, contributing to your overall well-being. By understanding the information presented on labels, you can select foods that align with the principles of an anti-inflammatory diet.

2.5. TIPS FOR GROCERY SHOPPING AND MEAL PLANNING

Efficient grocery shopping and thoughtful meal planning are pivotal aspects of embracing an anti-inflammatory lifestyle. These tips will guide beginners in making informed choices and cultivating a supportive culinary routine.

We'll provide practical guidance on navigating your grocery shopping endeavors, from formulating a comprehensive shopping list to making informed choices for optimal health. Meal planning is also a vital part of your anti-inflammatory journey. You'll learn how to plan your meals to ensure they're not only delicious but also inflammation-fighting powerhouses.

Example: Imagine shopping as a treasure hunt, with your list as your map. With our tips, you'll navigate the store like a seasoned explorer, finding treasures for your health.

A. GROCERY SHOPPING TIPS:

1. Prepare a Shopping List:
- Plan your meals in advance and create a detailed shopping list.
- Stick to the list to avoid impulsive purchases.

2. Shop the Perimeter:
- Whole, fresh foods like fruits, vegetables, and lean proteins are often located around the perimeter of the grocery store.
- Minimize processed foods found in the central aisles.

3. Choose Seasonal and Local Produce:
- Seasonal and local produce is often fresher and may have a higher nutrient content.
- Support local farmers and reduce environmental impact.

4. Read Labels Mindfully:
- Apply the knowledge from the section on "Navigating Food Labels" to make informed choices.
- Be discerning about ingredients and nutritional content.

5. Opt for Whole Foods:
- Prioritize whole, minimally processed foods.
- Select grains, nuts, and seeds in their unprocessed forms.

6. Buy in Bulk:
- Purchase staples like grains, legumes, and nuts in bulk to reduce packaging waste and save money.

7. Include a Variety of Colors:
- A colorful assortment of fruits and vegetables provides a range of nutrients.
- Aim for a diverse plate to support overall health.

B. MEAL PLANNING TIPS:

1. Plan Balanced Meals:
- Ensure each meal includes a variety of fruits, vegetables, lean proteins, and whole grains.
- Aim for a balance of macronutrients.

2. Batch Cooking:
- Cook larger quantities and freeze individual portions for convenient future meals.
- Saves time and encourages healthier eating habits.

3. Explore New Recipes:
- Keep your meals exciting by trying new anti-inflammatory recipes.
- Experiment with different ingredients and cooking techniques.

4. Prep Ingredients in Advance:
- Wash, chop, and portion ingredients ahead of time.
- Reduces preparation time during busy days.

5. Mindful Portion Control:
- Be conscious of portion sizes to avoid overeating.
- Use smaller plates to encourage appropriate portions.

6. Include Snacks:
- Plan for nutritious snacks to curb hunger between meals.
- Consider options like fresh fruit, veggies with hummus, or a handful of nuts.

7. Rotate Proteins:
- Vary protein sources to ensure a diverse nutrient intake.
- Include fish, poultry, plant-based proteins, and lean meats.

Upon concluding this chapter, you'll possess a solid understanding of the elements to incorporate and those to omit from your anti-inflammatory diet. Your visits to the grocery store will adopt a more deliberate purpose, and your meal planning will evolve into a harmonious blend of flavors and health advantages. It's a progression towards improved well-being, taking each bite with intention.

CHAPTER 3
EXERCISES TO REDUCE INFLAMMATION

3.1. INCORPORATING PHYSICAL ACTIVITY FOR BETTER HEALTH

Physical activity goes beyond mere weight loss or muscle building; it stands as a pivotal component of an anti-inflammatory way of life. It serves as a potent instrument in your repertoire to counter inflammation and enhance your overall well-being. Consistent engagement in physical activities contributes to the regulation of your immune system, improvement in blood circulation, and even a reduction in the levels of inflammatory markers within your body.

A. Understanding the Role of Physical Activity:
  - ➤ **Insight**: Physical activity is not only about weight management; it plays a crucial role in modulating inflammation.
  - ➤ **Example**: Regular exercise promotes the release of anti-inflammatory substances, contributing to overall well-being.

B. The Connection Between Exercise and Inflammation:

➢ **Correlation**: Engaging in physical activity has been linked to reduced levels of inflammatory markers in the body.

➢ **Illustration**: Studies suggest that regular exercise may help mitigate chronic inflammation associated with various health conditions.

C. Tailoring Your Fitness Routine to Combat Inflammation:

➢ **Personalization**: Your exercise routine can be tailored to address specific health concerns and target inflammatory pathways.

➢ **Example**: Incorporating both aerobic exercises and strength training can provide a comprehensive approach to inflammation reduction.

D. Yoga, Meditation, and Mindfulness for Stress Reduction:

➢ Holistic Approach: Practices like yoga and meditation not only improve flexibility and mental well-being but also help reduce stress-induced inflammation.

➤ Illustrative Instance: Mindful activities, such as deep breathing exercises, can have a calming effect on the body, influencing inflammatory responses.

E. Making Exercise Enjoyable:
➤ **Encouragement**: Choose activities you enjoy to make exercise a sustainable part of your routine.
➤ **Example**: Whether it's dancing, hiking, or playing a sport, finding joy in movement increases the likelihood of consistency.

F. Incorporating Movement Throughout the Day:
➤ **Practical Tips**: Small, frequent movements can add up. Break up long periods of sitting with short walks or stretching exercises.
➤ **Illustration**: Taking the stairs, stretching during work breaks, and opting for short walks contribute to overall physical activity.

G. Building a Balanced Exercise Routine:
➤ **Guidance**: Aim for a mix of cardiovascular exercises, strength training, and flexibility exercises for a well-rounded routine.

➢ **Example**: Cycling or brisk walking for cardiovascular health, strength training with weights, and yoga for flexibility create a comprehensive approach.

H. Progressing Gradually:

➢ **Caution**: If you're new to exercise, start gradually and listen to your body to avoid overexertion.

➢ **Illustrative Tip**: Begin with low-impact activities like walking and gradually increase intensity as your fitness level improves.

I. Social Engagement in Physical Activity:

➢ **Community Aspect**: Joining fitness classes or exercising with friends can provide motivation and make physical activity a social and enjoyable experience.

➢ **Example**: Participating in group activities like dance classes or hiking clubs fosters a sense of camaraderie.

Incorporating physical activity into your anti-inflammatory lifestyle is a powerful step towards holistic well-being. From personalized routines to enjoyable activities, finding ways to move your body contributes not only to reduced inflammation but also to increased vitality and overall health.

3.2. THE CONNECTION BETWEEN EXERCISE AND INFLAMMATION L

Comprehending the intricate interplay between exercise and inflammation proves paramount. While vigorous physical exertion may trigger transient inflammation, regular, moderate exercise demonstrates its effectiveness in mitigating chronic, low-grade inflammation. Achieving this delicate equilibrium is key. We will delve into the scientific intricacies of how exercise influences your immune system, elucidating its pivotal role in your journey toward an anti-inflammatory lifestyle.

Example: Consider exercise like a controlled burn in a forest. While it may spark a little inflammation initially, it clears the path for new growth and reduces the risk of catastrophic fires.

3.3. TAILORING YOUR FITNESS ROUTINE TO COMBAT INFLAMMATION

In the pursuit of an anti-inflammatory lifestyle, customizing your fitness routine is a key strategy to specifically target and reduce inflammation. Let's delve into the importance of tailoring your exercise regimen and explore practical examples to combat inflammation effectively.

A. Understanding Individual Health Needs:

➢ **Insight**: Consider your current health status and any existing inflammatory conditions when designing your fitness routine.

➢ **Example**: Individuals with arthritis may benefit from low-impact exercises like swimming or cycling to reduce joint stress.

B. Incorporating Cardiovascular Exercises:

➢ **Focus**: Cardiovascular exercises elevate heart rate and have a positive impact on inflammation markers.

➢ **Example**: Engage in activities like brisk walking, jogging, or cycling to enhance cardiovascular health and combat inflammation systemically.

C. Integrating Strength Training:

> **Importance**: Building muscle through strength training contributes to overall fitness and may help regulate inflammatory responses.

> **Example**: Include weightlifting, resistance band exercises, or bodyweight workouts to strengthen muscles and support inflammatory control.

D. Emphasizing Flexibility and Range of Motion:

> **Consideration**: Incorporate exercises that enhance flexibility, as improved range of motion can alleviate stiffness associated with inflammation.

> **Example**: Include yoga or Pilates in your routine to promote flexibility, balance, and joint mobility.

E. Interval Training for Metabolic Health:

> **Strategy**: High-intensity interval training (HIIT) has shown promise in improving metabolic health and regulating inflammation.

➢ **Example**: Integrate short bursts of intense exercise, like sprinting or jumping jacks, followed by periods of rest or lower-intensity activity.

F. Mind-Body Practices for Stress Reduction:
➢ **Holistic Approach:** Stress management is crucial in combating inflammation; incorporate mind-body practices.
➢ **Example**: Introduce mindfulness-based activities such as tai chi or qigong, which combine movement with meditation to reduce stress-induced inflammation.

G. Adapting to Personal Preferences:
➢ **Encouragement**: Choose activities that resonate with you to maintain consistency and enjoyment.
➢ **Example**: If you prefer outdoor activities, opt for hiking, gardening, or cycling to make exercise a fulfilling part of your routine.

H. Monitoring Intensity and Recovery:
➢ **Guidance**: Pay attention to exercise intensity to avoid overexertion, and allow adequate time for recovery.

➢ **Example**: Balance high-intensity workouts with lower-intensity sessions and prioritize recovery strategies like proper hydration and rest.

I. Consulting with Health Professionals:

➢ **Safety Measure**: If you have specific health concerns, consult with healthcare professionals or fitness experts to tailor your routine safely.

➢ **Example**: Individuals with chronic conditions like diabetes or heart disease may benefit from personalized advice to ensure exercise aligns with their health goals.

J. Tracking Progress and Adjusting:

➢ **Adaptability**: Regularly assess your fitness journey, track progress, and be open to adjusting your routine based on your evolving health needs.

➢ **Example**: If joint issues arise, modify exercises or explore alternatives to address concerns without compromising overall fitness.

Customizing your fitness routine to combat inflammation empowers you to address specific health goals and contribute to overall well-being. By tailoring exercises to your individual needs, you can create a sustainable and effective anti-inflammatory fitness plan that complements your journey towards a healthier lifestyle.

3.4. YOGA, MEDITATION, AND MINDFULNESS FOR STRESS REDUCTION

Stress acts as a notable contributor to inflammation, akin to fuel for the inflammatory fire. In this segment, we'll probe into how practices such as yoga, meditation, and mindfulness serve as effective tools for stress management. By mastering the art of relaxing both your mind and body, you can diminish chronic stress, which is a feeding ground for inflammation.

This chapter explores the profound impact of these mind-body activities on inflammation and provides practical examples for beginners looking to integrate them into their daily routine.

A. Yoga: Cultivating Harmony Between Body and Mind:

➤ **Purpose**: Yoga combines physical postures, breath control, and meditation to promote overall well-being.

➤ **Example**: Beginner-friendly yoga poses, such as Child's Pose or Downward Dog, can help release tension and foster a sense of calm.

B. Meditation: The Art of Cultivating Inner Stillness:

➤ **Focus**: Meditation involves training the mind to achieve a state of focused attention and relaxation.

➤ **Example**: Guided meditations or mindfulness apps can assist beginners in establishing a regular meditation practice.

C. Mindfulness: Present Moment Awareness for Stress Alleviation:

➤ Principle: Mindfulness emphasizes being fully present in the current moment without judgment.

➤ **Example**: Mindful eating, where you savor each bite, can transform a daily activity into a stress-relieving practice.

D. Yoga and Its Impact on Inflammation:

➢ **Connection**: Regular yoga practice has been linked to reduced levels of inflammatory markers in the body.

➢ **Example**: Sun Salutations, a dynamic series of poses, can enhance circulation and contribute to a sense of vitality.

E. Meditation's Influence on the Nervous System:

➢ **Benefit**: Meditation promotes relaxation, calming the sympathetic nervous system associated with stress.

➢ **Example**: Body Scan Meditation, focusing attention on each part of the body, helps release tension and induces a sense of calm.

F. Mindfulness for Stress Reduction:

➢ **Effectiveness**: Mindfulness practices contribute to stress reduction by fostering awareness and acceptance.

➢ **Example**: Engage in mindful breathing exercises, such as diaphragmatic breathing, to elicit the body's relaxation response.

G. Incorporating Mind-Body Practices Into Daily Routine:

> **Integration**: Seamlessly infuse these practices into daily activities, making them accessible for beginners.

> **Example:** Practice mindful walking by paying attention to each step and the sensations in your feet during a stroll.

H. Creating a Relaxing Yoga and Meditation Space:

> **Environment**: Dedicate a quiet space for yoga and meditation to enhance the calming effects.

> **Example**: Arrange cushions or a yoga mat in a well-lit area, creating a serene atmosphere for your practice.

I. Mindful Eating for Nutritional and Emotional Wellness:

> **Approach**: Mindful eating involves savoring each bite, promoting healthy digestion and a positive relationship with food.

> **Example**: During meals, focus on the flavors, textures, and sensations, fostering a mindful connection with nourishment.

J. Progressing Gradually in Mind-Body Practices:
> **Encouragement**: Begin with shorter sessions and gradually extend the duration to build a sustainable practice.
> **Example**: Start with 5–10 minutes of guided meditation or a gentle yoga routine, gradually increasing as you feel comfortable.

Incorporating yoga, meditation, and mindfulness into your anti-inflammatory lifestyle offers holistic benefits, promoting not only stress reduction but also contributing to overall well-being. By embracing these practices, beginners can create a foundation for a more balanced and mindful approach to daily life.

This chapter extends beyond the realm of perspiration; it's about comprehending the profound influence that exercise and stress management wield over your body's inflammatory response. It stands as a vital piece in the anti-inflammatory puzzle, and as you conclude this chapter, you'll be well-prepared to seamlessly integrate exercise and relaxation practices into your daily routine.

CHAPTER 4
ANTI-INFLAMMATORY COOKING BASICS

4.1. ESTABLISHING YOUR KITCHEN FOR AN ANTI-INFLAMMATORY CULINARY EXPERIENCE

Your kitchen is your battleground against inflammation, and it's essential to set it up for success. Within this segment, we'll provide detailed instructions on establishing a kitchen conducive to anti-inflammatory practices.

Example: Your kitchen is like an artist's studio. By having a well-organized palette of anti-inflammatory ingredients and the right tools, you can create masterpieces of health and flavor.

Setting up your kitchen to align with an anti-inflammatory culinary experience is a foundational step in embracing a healthier lifestyle. This chapter provides guidance on creating an environment that supports anti-inflammatory cooking, offering practical examples for beginners to cultivate a kitchen conducive to their well-being.

A. Stocking Anti-Inflammatory Ingredients:

➤ **Essentials**: Fill your pantry with staples like whole grains, legumes, nuts, seeds, and a variety of colorful fruits and vegetables.

➤ **Example**: Keep quinoa, lentils, walnuts, chia seeds, and a rainbow of fresh produce readily available for versatile and nutritious meal preparation.

B. Embracing Fresh and Seasonal Produce:

➤ **Strategy**: Prioritize fresh, seasonal fruits and vegetables to maximize nutrient content and flavor.

➤ **Example**: During summer, incorporate berries, tomatoes, and leafy greens, while opting for root vegetables and citrus fruits in the colder months.

C. Opting for Whole, Unprocessed Foods:

➤ **Principle**: Choose whole foods over processed alternatives to minimize additives and maximize nutritional benefits.

➤ **Example**: Instead of packaged snacks, reach for whole fruits, raw nuts, or homemade energy bites for a satisfying and nourishing treat.

D. Exploring a Variety of Herbs and Spices:
- ➢ **Versatility**: Enhance flavors without relying on excess salt or sugar by incorporating a diverse range of herbs and spices.
- ➢ **Example**: Experiment with turmeric, ginger, garlic, basil, and cilantro to elevate the taste profile of your dishes while reaping their anti-inflammatory properties.

E. Choosing Healthy Fats and Oils:
- ➢ **Selection**: Opt for heart-healthy fats like olive oil, avocado oil, and omega-3-rich sources such as flaxseed oil.
- ➢ **Example**: Use olive oil for salad dressings and sautéing, and drizzle flaxseed oil over dishes for an added nutritional boost.

F. Mindful Grocery Shopping for Quality Ingredients:
- ➢ **Approach**: Read labels, choose organic when possible, and prioritize high-quality ingredients to enhance the nutritional value of your meals.
- ➢ **Example**: Select organic, grass-fed meats or wild-caught fish to minimize exposure to additives and maximize nutrient content.

G. Investing in Kitchen Tools for Efficiency:

➢ **Essentials**: Acquire tools such as a high-quality knife, cutting board, blender, and food processor to streamline your cooking process.

➢ **Example**: A sharp chef's knife facilitates precise chopping, while a blender is perfect for creating nutrient-packed smoothies or soups.

H. Organizing Your Kitchen for Accessibility:

➢ **Efficiency**: Arrange your kitchen to make frequently used items easily accessible, promoting a seamless cooking experience.

➢ **Example**: Keep commonly used spices within reach, organize pantry items logically, and designate a space for fresh produce in the refrigerator.

I. Minimizing Processed and Sugary Ingredients:

➢ **Guideline**: Reduce reliance on processed foods and limit added sugars to align with anti-inflammatory principles.

➢ **Example**: Instead of sugary sauces, prepare homemade versions using fresh tomatoes, herbs, and a touch of natural sweetness from ingredients like balsamic vinegar.

J. Building a Sustainable Meal Prep Routine:
➢ **Planning**: Dedicate time for weekly meal prep to streamline cooking, ensuring nutritious meals are readily available.
➢ **Example**: Chop vegetables in advance, cook batches of grains, and marinate proteins for quick and convenient assembling during the week.

By establishing a kitchen that prioritizes anti-inflammatory ingredients and efficient cooking practices, beginners can create a supportive environment for their culinary journey. This approach not only enhances the nutritional quality of meals but also makes the process enjoyable and sustainable for long-term well-being.

4.2. MASTERING COOKING APPROACHES IN LINE WITH AN ANTI-INFLAMMATORY EATING PLAN

Culinary endeavors transcend mere food preparation; they embody both an art and a science. In this section of the chapter, we'll delve into diverse culinary techniques that harmonize with an anti-inflammatory dietary regimen. You'll discover methods that help preserve the nutritional value of your ingredients while reducing the formation of harmful compounds. From steaming and sautéing to roasting and grilling, we'll provide you with a toolkit of cooking techniques to enhance your meals.

Cooking techniques are like different brushstrokes on a canvas. Each technique adds depth and character to your culinary creations, ensuring they are not only delicious but also health-enhancing.

A. Sautéing with Healthy Oils:
- ➤ **Technique**: Use minimal oil and opt for heart-healthy choices like olive oil or coconut oil for sautéing.
- ➤ Example: Sautéing vegetables in olive oil with garlic and herbs enhances flavor without compromising the nutritional value.

B. Steaming for Nutrient Retention:
- ➤ **Approach**: Steam vegetables to preserve their vitamins and minerals that may be lost through boiling.
- ➤ **Example**: Steamed broccoli or asparagus retains vibrant colors and optimal nutritional content.

C. Grilling for Flavorful Options:
- ➤ **Method**: Grill lean proteins, vegetables, and fruits for a smoky flavor without excessive added fats.
- ➤ **Example**: Grilled chicken or vegetable skewers with a marinade of herbs and citrus offer a delicious and anti-inflammatory option.

D. Roasting to Enhance Natural Flavors:
- ➤ **Technique**: Roast vegetables and proteins to intensify their natural sweetness and create depth of flavor.
- ➤ **Example**: Roasted sweet potatoes with a sprinkle of cinnamon and rosemary provide a nutrient-rich side dish.

E. Baking with Whole Ingredients:

➢ **Approach**: Opt for baking as a method to create wholesome dishes using whole grains, nuts, and fruits.

➢ **Example**: Baked oatmeal with berries and nuts combines fiber and antioxidants for a nourishing breakfast.

F. Poaching for Delicate Preparation:

➢ **Method**: Poach proteins such as fish or chicken in flavorful liquids to maintain moisture without excess fats.

➢ **Example**: Poached salmon in a broth of herbs and lemon ensures a tender and heart-healthy main course.

G. Stir-Frying with Colorful Vegetables:

➢ **Technique**: Quickly stir-fry vegetables at high heat to retain their vibrant colors and crisp texture.

➢ **Example**: Stir-fried rainbow vegetables with tofu or lean protein offer a visually appealing and nutritious meal.

H. Raw Preparations for Freshness:

➢ **Approach**: Incorporate raw elements like salads or smoothies to maximize the intake of enzymes and nutrients.

➢ **Example**: A refreshing salad with a variety of leafy greens, colorful vegetables, and a homemade vinaigrette provides a raw and nutrient-packed meal.

I. Slow Cooking for Tender Results:

➢ **Method**: Utilize a slow cooker for hands-off cooking that yields tender and flavorful dishes.

➢ **Example**: Slow-cooked chili with lean meats, beans, and a medley of spices ensures a comforting and anti-inflammatory meal.

J. Herbs and Spices for Flavor Enhancement:

➢ **Enhancement**: Experiment with a variety of herbs and spices to elevate flavors without relying on excessive salt or sugar.

➢ **Example**: Marinating proteins with a blend of turmeric, cumin, and coriander adds depth and anti-inflammatory benefits.

By mastering these cooking approaches in line with an anti-inflammatory eating plan, beginners can not only create delicious meals but also amplify the health benefits of their culinary creations. Experimenting with these techniques allows for a diverse and enjoyable anti-inflammatory cooking experience.

4.3. MAXIMIZING THE POTENTIAL OF HERBS AND SPICES TO ENHANCE TASTE AND WELL-BEING

Herbs and spices serve as the clandestine champions in the realm of anti-inflammatory cuisine. Beyond imparting richness and zest to your culinary creations, they unveil a treasure trove of health advantages. Join us as we embark on an exploration of the diverse universe of herbs and spices, unraveling their distinct anti-inflammatory attributes and guiding you on seamlessly integrating them into your gastronomic endeavors. From turmeric and ginger to rosemary and garlic, you'll grasp the art of infusing your meals with both palatability and well-being.

Example: Think of herbs and spices as the artists' colors on your culinary canvas. Each one brings its own vibrancy and depth to your dishes, creating a masterpiece of flavor and health.

A. Turmeric:
- Flavor Profile: Earthy and slightly bitter.
- Health Benefits: Contains curcumin, known for its anti-inflammatory and antioxidant properties.

Example: Golden turmeric latte with almond milk and a pinch of black pepper.

B. Ginger:
- Flavor Profile: Spicy and zesty.
- Health Benefits: Anti-inflammatory and aids digestion.

Example: Ginger-infused green tea for a soothing and health-boosting beverage.

C. Garlic:
- Flavor Profile: Pungent and savory.
- Health Benefits: Exhibits anti-inflammatory and immune-boosting properties.

Example: Roasted garlic mashed sweet potatoes for a flavorful and nutritious side dish.

D. Cinnamon:
- Flavor Profile: Sweet and warm.
- Health Benefits: Anti-inflammatory and may help regulate blood sugar.

Example: Cinnamon-spiced overnight oats for a delicious and health-conscious breakfast.

E. Rosemary:
- Flavor Profile: Woody and aromatic.
- Health Benefits: Contains antioxidants and anti-inflammatory compounds.

Example: Grilled rosemary-infused chicken for a fragrant and savory main course.

F. Basil:
- Flavor Profile: Sweet and slightly peppery.
- Health Benefits: Anti-inflammatory and rich in vitamins.

Example: Fresh basil pesto with whole grain pasta for a vibrant and nutrient-packed meal.

G. Cumin:
- Flavor Profile: Earthy and warm.
- Health Benefits: Anti-inflammatory and aids digestion.

Example: Cumin-spiced roasted chickpeas as a crunchy and nutritious snack.

H. Coriander:
- Flavor Profile: Citrusy and slightly sweet.
- Health Benefits: Anti-inflammatory and rich in antioxidants.

Example: Coriander-spiced quinoa salad for a refreshing and healthful side dish.

I. Oregano:
- Flavor Profile: Robust and slightly bitter.
- Health Benefits: Contains antimicrobial and anti-inflammatory properties.

Example: Greek-style oregano-infused roasted vegetables for a flavorful and nutritious medley.

J. Mint:
- Flavor Profile: Refreshing and cool.
- Health Benefits: Aids digestion and may have calming effects.

Example: Mint-infused fruit salad for a refreshing and digestive-friendly dessert.

Experimenting with these herbs and spices not only adds depth and complexity to dishes but also infuses them with health-promoting compounds. By maximizing the potential of herbs and spices in their anti-inflammatory cooking journey, beginners can create meals that are both delicious and supportive of overall well-being.

4.4. HEALTHY OILS AND FATS:
COOKING ESSENTIALS

In an anti-inflammatory diet, fats aren't adversaries; the emphasis lies in making discerning choices. Within this segment, we'll traverse the landscape of healthful oils and fats. You'll acquaint yourself with the optimal cooking oils for various dishes and glean insights on their effective utilization. From extra virgin olive oil to avocado oil, these fats not only elevate the taste of your culinary creations but also actively contribute to diminishing inflammation.

Here are key elements to consider:

A. Olive Oil:
- Type: Extra virgin olive oil.
- Health Benefits: Rich in monounsaturated fats and antioxidants.
- Usage: Drizzling over salads or using in sautéing for a Mediterranean touch.

Example: Caprese salad with extra virgin olive oil for a light and flavorful dish.

B. Coconut Oil:
- Type: Unrefined, virgin coconut oil.
- Health Benefits: Contains medium-chain triglycerides (MCTs) with potential health benefits.
- Usage: Ideal for baking, stir-frying, or adding a subtle coconut flavor to dishes.

Example: Coconut oil-infused sweet potato fries for a tasty and nutritious snack.

C. Avocado:
- Type: Whole avocados or avocado oil.
- Health Benefits: Packed with heart-healthy monounsaturated fats.
- Usage: Perfect for salads, dips, or as a finishing touch on cooked dishes.

Example: Avocado and black bean salad with a lime and avocado oil dressing for a creamy and nutritious meal.

D. Flaxseed Oil:
- Type: Cold-pressed flaxseed oil.
- Health Benefits: High in omega-3 fatty acids, known for anti-inflammatory properties.

- Usage: Use as a salad dressing or drizzle on dishes after cooking.

Example: Quinoa and vegetable bowl with flaxseed oil vinaigrette for a nourishing and omega-3-rich meal.

E. Walnut Oil:
- Type: Cold-pressed walnut oil.
- Health Benefits: Contains omega-3 fatty acids and antioxidants.
- Usage: Ideal for drizzling over salads or incorporating into dressings.

Example: Mixed greens with pear and goat cheese drizzled with walnut oil for a nutty and flavorful salad.

F. Ghee:
- Type: Clarified butter.
- Health Benefits: Lactose-free and rich in fat-soluble vitamins.
- Usage: Suitable for sautéing or as a substitute for butter in various recipes.

Example: Sautéed vegetables in ghee with a hint of turmeric for a golden and savory side dish.

G. Salmon and Fatty Fish:

- Source: Fatty fish like salmon, mackerel, and sardines.
- Health Benefits: High in omega-3 fatty acids.
- Usage: Grilled or baked for a delicious and heart-healthy main course.

Example: Baked salmon with lemon and herbs for a flavorful and omega-3-rich dish.

H. Nuts and Seeds:

- Sources: Almonds, chia seeds, and sunflower seeds.
- Health Benefits: Provide healthy fats, fiber, and various nutrients.
- Usage: Sprinkle on salads, yogurt, or incorporate into smoothies.

Example: Greek yogurt parfait with almonds and chia seeds for a crunchy and nutritious dessert.

I. Dark Chocolate:
- Type: High-quality dark chocolate with at least 70% cocoa.
- Health Benefits: Contains antioxidants and may have anti-inflammatory effects.
- Usage: Enjoyed in moderation as a delightful treat.

Example: Dark chocolate-dipped strawberries for a decadent and antioxidant-rich dessert.

J. Seed Butters:
- Sources: Almond butter or tahini (sesame seed butter).
- Health Benefits: Provide healthy fats and are versatile in various dishes.
- Usage: Spread on whole-grain toast, blend into smoothies, or use in dressings.

Example: Almond butter and banana sandwich on whole-grain bread for a satisfying and nutritious snack.

By incorporating these healthy oils and fats into their cooking repertoire, beginners can not only enhance the taste of their dishes but also support their overall well-being on their anti-inflammatory journey.

Upon concluding this chapter, your kitchen will undergo a metamorphosis into a sanctuary of anti-inflammatory culinary ingenuity. Armed with knowledge and culinary tools, you'll be adept at crafting meals that not only tantalize the taste buds but also foster health. These foundational cooking principles stand as the cornerstone of your journey toward an anti-inflammatory lifestyle, enabling you to relish the flavors of well-being in every morsel.

CHAPTER 5
60-DAY MEAL PLAN

5.1. CREATING A SUSTAINABLE ANTI-INFLAMMATORY MEAL PLAN

Initiating an anti-inflammatory expedition extends beyond singular recipes; it entails formulating a sustainable and comprehensive dietary strategy. Within this segment, we'll steer you through the intricacies of developing an anti-inflammatory meal plan tailored to align with your lifestyle. We'll aid you in establishing pragmatic objectives, ensuring that your meal plan not only prioritizes health but also remains gratifying and enduring in the long run.

Envision your meal plan as a navigational guide for your anti-inflammatory odyssey. It should lead you to a destination of better health, filled with delicious stops along the way.

A. Balanced Nutrient Intake:
> **Principle**: Ensure a well-rounded mix of macronutrients – carbohydrates, proteins, and healthy fats – to provide sustained energy and nourishment.

- **Example**: Quinoa salad with chickpeas, vegetables, and a drizzle of olive oil, offering a balance of protein, fiber, and healthy fats.

B. Incorporate a Rainbow of Vegetables:
➢ **Principle**: Include a variety of colorful vegetables to access a spectrum of nutrients and antioxidants.
- **Example**: Roasted vegetable medley with bell peppers, carrots, broccoli, and sweet potatoes, offering a diverse range of vitamins and minerals.

C. Lean Protein Sources:
➢ **Principle**: Opt for lean protein sources like fish, poultry, tofu, or legumes to support muscle health without excessive saturated fats.
- **Example**: Grilled salmon with quinoa and steamed asparagus, providing omega-3 fatty acids and complete proteins.

D. Incorporate Whole Grains:
➢ **Principle**: Choose whole grains over refined options for added fiber, vitamins, and minerals.

- **Example**: Brown rice bowl with black beans, sautéed greens, and a sprinkle of seeds, offering a nutrient-dense and filling meal.

E. Healthy Fats in Moderation:
➢ **Principle**: Include sources of healthy fats, such as avocados, nuts, and olive oil, in moderation to support overall well-being.
- **Example**: Avocado and walnut salad with a light vinaigrette, providing a mix of monounsaturated fats and antioxidants.

F. Mindful Portion Control:
➢ **Principle**: Practice mindful eating and portion control to maintain a healthy weight and prevent overconsumption.
- **Example**: Savoring a small serving of dark chocolate as a dessert rather than indulging in excessive amounts.

G. Hydration is Key:
➢ **Principle**: Stay adequately hydrated with water, herbal teas, and infused water to support overall health.
- **Example**: Infused cucumber and mint water as a refreshing and hydrating beverage.

H. Variety and Adaptability:

➢ **Principle**: Embrace a variety of foods and be adaptable to seasonal produce for freshness and diversity.

- **Example**: Adjusting recipes based on seasonal vegetables, incorporating freshness and supporting local produce.

I. Meal Prep and Batch Cooking:

➢ **Principle**: Plan and prepare meals in advance to save time and ensure adherence to the anti-inflammatory diet.

- **Example**: Preparing a batch of vegetable and lentil soup for the week, promoting convenience and adherence to the meal plan.

J. Flexibility for Dining Out:

➢ **Principle**: Maintain flexibility for social occasions and dining out while making mindful choices.

- **Example**: Choosing grilled fish with a side of steamed vegetables when dining at a restaurant, aligning with the anti-inflammatory principles.

Creating a sustainable anti-inflammatory meal plan involves incorporating these principles into daily eating habits, fostering not only health but also a sustainable and enjoyable culinary journey for beginners.

5.2. WEEK-BY-WEEK MEAL PLANS WITH DAILY RECIPES

We understand that planning meals can be a daunting task. This is precisely why we have meticulously crafted meal plans structured on a week-by-week basis, accompanied by daily recipes. These meticulously designed plans aim to eliminate any uncertainties surrounding your meals, offering you a distinct and straightforward route to follow. Every week is thoughtfully arranged to present a diverse array of flavors while ensuring that you reap the anti-inflammatory advantages you are striving for.

WEEK 1: Introduction to Anti-Inflammatory Basics
Day 1:

- ➤ **Breakfast**: Berry and Spinach Smoothie with Chia Seeds
- ➤ **Lunch**: Quinoa Salad with Grilled Chicken and Avocado
- ➤ **Dinner**: Baked Salmon with Lemon and Herb Quinoa.

Day 2:

- ➤ **Breakfast**: Greek Yogurt Parfait with Mixed Berries and Almonds
- ➤ **Lunch**: Lentil and Vegetable Soup
- ➤ **Dinner**: Stir-Fried Tofu with Broccoli and Brown Rice

Day 3:

- ➤ **Breakfast**: Oatmeal with Sliced Banana and Walnuts
- ➤ **Lunch**: Chickpea Salad with Cucumber and Feta
- ➤ **Dinner**: Grilled Turkey Burgers with Sweet Potato Fries.

WEEK 2: Exploring Culinary Diversity

Day 1:
- ➤ **Breakfast**: Mango and Coconut Milk Smoothie Bowl
- ➤ **Lunch**: Spinach and Feta Stuffed Bell Peppers
- ➤ **Dinner**: Baked Cod with Tomato and Olive Relish.

Day 2:
- ➤ **Breakfast**: Whole Grain Toast with Avocado and Poached Egg.
- ➤ **Lunch**: Quinoa and Black Bean Bowl with Lime Vinaigrette.
- ➤ **Dinner**: Vegetable Stir-Fry with Shrimp and Quinoa.

Day 3:
- ➤ **Breakfast**: Blueberry and Almond Butter Overnight Oats
- ➤ **Lunch**: Greek Chicken Salad with Tzatziki Dressing
- ➤ **Dinner**: Lentil and Vegetable Curry with Brown Rice.

WEEK 3: Embracing Seasonal Ingredients

Day 1:

- ➤ **Breakfast**: Peach and Raspberry Smoothie
- ➤ **Lunch**: Roasted Butternut Squash and Kale Salad
- ➤ **Dinner**: Grilled Chicken with Mango Salsa and Wild Rice

Day 2:

- ➤ Breakfast: Apple and Cinnamon Chia Seed Pudding.
- ➤ Lunch: Tomato and Basil Quinoa Bowl
- ➤ Dinner: Baked Halibut with Asparagus and Lemon

Day 3:

- ➤ Breakfast: Pumpkin Spice Overnight Oats
- ➤ Lunch: Brussels Sprouts and Pomegranate Salad.
- ➤ Dinner: Turkey and Vegetable Skewers with Quinoa.

Each week introduces new recipes and flavors, ensuring a diverse and enjoyable anti-inflammatory culinary experience for beginners. The meal plans focus on accessibility, nutrition, and simplicity, making the transition to an anti-inflammatory diet a delightful journey.

5.3. TIPS FOR SUCCESSFUL MEAL PLANNING AND PREPARATION

Achieving success in meal planning encompasses more than merely selecting recipes; it involves streamlined and effective preparation. Within this guide, we'll furnish you with invaluable insights and strategies to streamline your meal planning and preparation processes, making the entire experience effortless. From creating shopping lists to organizing your kitchen and cooking in batches, these strategies will streamline your anti-inflammatory cooking process.

Here are practical tips for beginners to ensure successful implementation of their anti-inflammatory culinary adventure:

1. Create a Weekly Meal Plan:

Plan your meals for the week, considering a balance of protein, vegetables, healthy fats, and whole grains.

2. Batch Cooking for Efficiency:

Prepare large batches of staples like quinoa, roasted vegetables, and lean proteins to use in various meals throughout the week.

3. Prep Ingredients in Advance:

Wash, chop, and portion vegetables and fruits on the weekend, making it easier to assemble meals during busy weekdays.

4. Embrace Freezer-Friendly Options:

Cook and freeze portions of soups, stews, and casseroles for quick and nutritious meals on hectic days.

5. Utilize Mason Jar Salads:

Layer salads in mason jars, starting with dressing at the bottom, followed by hearty vegetables, proteins, and greens on top, ensuring freshness until consumption.

6. Incorporate One-Pan Recipes:

Opt for recipes that require minimal cleanup, such as sheet pan dinners or one-pot meals, saving time and effort.

7. Experiment with Spice Blends:

Create custom spice blends to add flavor without relying on excess salt, sugar, or processed condiments.

8. Mindful Portion Control:

Use smaller plates to encourage portion control and prevent overeating, promoting a balanced intake of nutrients.

9. Stay Organized with a Grocery List:

Plan your grocery list based on your weekly meal plan to avoid impulse purchases and ensure you have all necessary ingredients.

10. Explore New Recipes Regularly:

Challenge yourself to try one new anti-inflammatory recipe each week to keep your meals exciting and diversified.

11. Rotate Protein Sources:

Vary your protein intake by including sources like fish, poultry, beans, and tofu to ensure a diverse nutrient profile.

12. Prep Smoothie Ingredients in Advance:

Portion smoothie ingredients, like fruits and greens, into individual bags and store them in the freezer for quick and convenient morning smoothies.

13. Invest in Quality Storage Containers:

Use glass or BPA-free plastic containers to store prepped ingredients and leftovers safely.

14. Plan for Flexibility:

Have a selection of quick and simple recipes for busy days and more elaborate options for when you have more time to enjoy the cooking process.

By incorporating these tips into their routine, beginners can efficiently plan and prepare anti-inflammatory meals, making the dietary transition enjoyable, sustainable, and conducive to overall well-being.

5.4. BATCH COOKING AND MEAL PREPPING STRATEGIES

Effective batch cooking and meal prepping play pivotal roles in a successful journey toward an anti-inflammatory culinary lifestyle. These approaches not only save valuable time but also guarantee that nourishing meals are readily accessible. Below are practical insights and illustrations for novices looking to adeptly navigate the realms of batch cooking and meal prepping:

1. Select Adaptable Ingredients:

Opt for ingredients such as quinoa, sweet potatoes, and lean proteins that offer versatility across a range of dishes throughout the week.

2. Dedicated Sunday Prep Sessions:

Allocate a few hours every Sunday to prepare fundamental items like brown rice, grilled chicken, and roasted vegetables, establishing a foundation for the upcoming week.

3. Employ a Divide-and-Conquer Approach:

Cook proteins separately from vegetables to uphold their distinct flavors and textures, fostering a variety of meal combinations.

4. Harness the Power of Slow Cookers and Instant Pots:

Craft hearty stews or soups using a slow cooker or Instant Pot, facilitating hands-free cooking and yielding multiple portions.

5. Exercise Portion Control with Containers:

Invest in containers of appropriate sizes to partition meals, averting overindulgence and simplifying the reheating process.

6. Freeze in Individual Servings:

Distribute soups, sauces, or casseroles into individual containers and freeze them, ensuring a diverse array of convenient, ready-to-consume options.

7. Label and Date Items:

Attach labels to containers indicating the preparation date and contents, enabling freshness tracking and minimizing food wastage.

8. Create Do-It-Yourself Freezer Packs:

Assemble freezer packs featuring pre-cut vegetables, protein, and seasonings for swift stir-fries or effortless sheet pan dinners.

9. Prepare Components, Not Just Full Meals:

Dice vegetables, marinate proteins, and measure out spices, streamlining the cooking process throughout the week.

10. Consider Preparing Double Batches:

When executing a recipe, contemplate making a double batch and freezing half for future use, saving time during busier days.

11. Plan for Mix-and-Match Meals:

Prepare an assortment of proteins, grains, and vegetables, providing flexibility to mix and match components for diverse meals.

12. Mindful Storage of Fresh Produce:

Preserve the freshness of produce by storing them appropriately, employing techniques like storing herbs with damp paper towels or using crispers for vegetables.

13. Theme-Based Meal Prepping:

Devise meal prepping sessions with thematic elements, such as a Mexican-inspired session featuring lean ground turkey, black beans, and salsa for various dishes.

14. Creatively Repurpose Leftovers:

Transform roasted vegetables into a nourishing grain bowl, or repurpose leftover grilled chicken as a delightful topping for a vibrant salad, minimizing food waste.

15. Rotate Flavors and Cuisines:

Explore diverse flavor profiles and cuisines on a weekly basis to keep meals enticing and prevent palate fatigue.

By integrating these batch cooking and meal prepping strategies, newcomers can adeptly prepare and savor anti-inflammatory meals, ensuring a continuous supply of wholesome and flavorsome options throughout the week.

5.5. EATING OUT AND STAYING ON TRACK

Eating out doesn't mean you have to deviate from your anti-inflammatory plan. We'll provide you with the information and tactics necessary to make discerning decisions while dining at restaurants or opting for takeout. You'll gain insights into effectively perusing menus, posing inquiries about ingredients, and adhering to your dietary goals even when you find yourself outside the confines of your personal kitchen.

Eating out can be like exploring new horizons. With the right guidance, you can continue your anti-inflammatory journey while savoring flavors from around the world.

Here are practical suggestions and instances to assist you in staying on course when enjoying meals outside:

1. **Examine the Menu in Advance:**
   Scrutinize the restaurant's menu online before venturing out, searching for dishes abundant in anti-inflammatory components such as vegetables, lean proteins, and whole grains.

2. Select Grilled or Roasted Proteins:

Favor grilled or roasted selections over fried ones. For instance, a grilled chicken breast or roasted fish can serve as commendable anti-inflammatory choices.

3. Embrace Vegetables:

Prioritize dishes centered around vegetables or salads. For example, a vibrant salad with leafy greens, tomatoes, and avocado can be both delectable and anti-inflammatory.

4. Opt for Whole Grains:

Choose whole grains like quinoa or brown rice when they are on the menu. These grains provide fiber and essential nutrients, contributing to an anti-inflammatory dietary approach.

5. Conscious Choices with Sauces and Dressings:

Request sauces and dressings on the side. This approach allows you to regulate the amount you use, avoiding excessive intake of added sugars or unhealthy fats.

6. Explore with Herbs and Spices:

Elevate your meal's flavor with herbs and spices rather than relying on salt or heavy sauces. For instance, inquire about dishes seasoned with turmeric, garlic, or ginger.

7. Personalize Your Order:

Feel empowered to modify your order based on your preferences and dietary requirements. Don't hesitate to ask for substitutions or adjustments aligning with anti-inflammatory choices.

8. Monitor Portion Sizes:

Be mindful of portion sizes, and contemplate sharing dishes or taking leftovers home. This practice aids in preventing overeating and promotes balanced consumption.

9. Stay Hydrated with Water or Herbal Tea:

Opt for water or herbal tea instead of sugary beverages. Adequate hydration is vital for overall health and complements an anti-inflammatory lifestyle.

10. Exercise Caution with Desserts:

If you indulge in dessert, opt for choices with less refined sugar. Fresh fruit, sorbet, or a modest serving of dark chocolate can be gratifying yet mindful selections.

11. Inquire and Communicate:

Feel at ease asking the server about preparation methods or dish ingredients. Clear communication ensures your dietary preferences are accommodated.

12. Prioritize a Stress-Free Dining Setting:

Choose a comfortable environment for your meal. Stress can contribute to inflammation, so curating a relaxed dining experience is advantageous.

13. Share Socially:

Communicate your anti-inflammatory journey with dining companions. This fosters understanding and support, enhancing the dining experience for everyone.

14. Embrace Moderation:

Relish your meal mindfully, savoring each bite. Moderation is pivotal in maintaining an anti-inflammatory equilibrium, even when dining out.

By adopting these strategies, beginners can navigate restaurant choices with confidence while remaining devoted to an anti-inflammatory lifestyle. Dining out can be a pleasurable experience that aligns harmoniously with your health objectives.

This chapter is your roadmap to the practical aspects of anti-inflammatory eating. With a sustainable meal plan, daily recipes, preparation tips, and strategies for dining out, you'll be well-prepared to embark on your 60-day anti-inflammatory journey. It's a journey towards better health and a more vibrant you, one meal at a time.

CHAPTER 6
RECIPES BY CATEGORY

In this chapter, we invite you to explore a treasure trove of anti-inflammatory recipes, organized into ten distinct categories to suit your every culinary need.

★ SECTION 1: BREAKFAST RECIPES
A Variety of Healthy Morning Options

Initiate your day with an assortment of breakfast recipes that not only tantalize your taste buds but also boast anti-inflammatory properties. Ranging from substantial oatmeal adorned with berries abundant in antioxidants to protein-rich smoothie bowls, you'll encounter choices that transform your mornings into a jubilation of well-being.
enance while adhering to an anti-inflammatory lifestyle.

★ BREAKFAST RECIPES :

1. Radiant Turmeric Smoothie:
An energetic and anti-inflammatory fusion of turmeric, ginger, banana, and almond milk to commence your day with a brilliant burst of goodness.

2. Quinoa Morning Bowl:

Brimming with protein, this quinoa bowl showcases fresh berries, nuts, and a drizzle of honey, presenting a delightful and satiating breakfast alternative.

3. Avocado Toast with Poached Egg:

A contemporary classic elevated – whole grain toast crowned with velvety avocado, a flawlessly poached egg, and a sprinkling of inflammation-taming herbs.

4. Assorted Berry Chia Pudding:

A charming chia seed pudding infused with an assortment of berries, delivering a surge of antioxidants and omega-3 fatty acids.

5. Anti-Inflammatory Smoothie Bowl:

A vibrant bowl featuring berries, spinach, and omega-3-rich seeds, blended into a smooth and revitalizing bowl of wholesomeness.

6. Sweet Potato and Spinach Breakfast Frittata:

A savory frittata packed with sweet potatoes, spinach, and herbs, providing a flavorsome and anti-inflammatory twist to your breakfast ritual.

7. Oatmeal with Almond Butter and Berries:

Creamy oatmeal crowned with a dollop of almond butter and a scattering of fresh berries, delivering a hearty and gratifying breakfast.

8. Coconut Yogurt Parfait:

Layers of coconut yogurt, granola, and fresh fruits, crafting a delectable parfait that's not only delightful but also anti-inflammatory.

Each recipe is meticulously designed to ignite your mornings with a fusion of taste and health. Embrace the assortment, relish the flavors, and commence your day with breakfasts that contribute to your anti-inflammatory journey.

★ SECTION 2: SALAD RECIPES

Nutrient-Packed Salad Ideas

Welcome to the second section of the *Anti-Inflammatory Cookbook for Beginners*, where we embark on a flavorful exploration of nutrient-packed salad recipes. These salads are not only a feast for the taste buds but are also designed to align seamlessly with your anti-inflammatory lifestyle. Let's dive into a world of vibrant ingredients and wholesome flavors.

★ SALAD RECIPES:

1. Quinoa and Kale Power Salad:

A hearty combination of quinoa, nutrient-rich kale, cherry tomatoes, and a lemon-tahini dressing, providing a powerful start to your anti-inflammatory journey.

2. Berry and Walnut Spinach Salad:

A refreshing spinach salad featuring a medley of berries, crunchy walnuts, and a balsamic vinaigrette, delivering a delightful burst of antioxidants.

3. Citrus Shrimp Avocado Bowl:

A zesty salad with succulent shrimp, creamy avocado, citrus segments, and mixed greens, creating a light yet satisfying dish rich in anti-inflammatory goodness.

4. Mango Tango Chicken Salad:

A tropical-inspired salad with grilled chicken, fresh mango, mixed greens, and a cilantro-lime dressing, infusing your mealtime with a dance of flavors and health benefits.

5. Roasted Cauliflower Lentil Salad:

A warm salad featuring roasted cauliflower, protein-packed lentils, cherry tomatoes, and a turmeric-infused dressing, offering a comforting and nutritious option.

6. Greek Quinoa Salad with Feta:

A Greek-inspired quinoa salad complete with tomatoes, cucumbers, olives, and feta cheese, tossed in a lemon-oregano dressing for a Mediterranean delight.

7. Salmon and Avocado Spring Mix:

A protein-rich salad combining flaky salmon, creamy avocado, mixed spring greens, and a ginger-soy dressing, bringing a touch of elegance to your anti-inflammatory plate.

8. Pomegranate Walnut Beet Salad:

A vibrant salad featuring roasted beets, juicy pomegranate seeds, walnuts, and arugula, drizzled with a honey-balsamic vinaigrette, adding a symphony of colors and textures to your meal.

These nutrient-packed salad ideas are crafted to elevate your dining experience while supporting your anti-inflammatory goals. Embrace the diversity of flavors, revel in the freshness, and let these salads be a delightful and healthful addition to your anti-inflammatory culinary journey.

★ SECTION 3: FISH AND SEAFOOD RECIPES

Delicious Seafood Dishes

Welcome to the third segment of the **"Anti-Inflammatory Cookbook for Beginners"**, where we plunge into a luscious selection of marine delights. These concoctions are meticulously fashioned not just to excite your palate but to seamlessly harmonize with your anti-inflammatory dietary path. Let's delve into the profound dimensions of taste and well-being that seafood can grace upon your dining tableau.

★ FISH AND SEAFOOD RECIPES

1. Citrus-Infused Grilled Salmon:

Salmon artfully grilled, bathed in the vibrant essences of citrus and garlic, crafting a succulent, rich dish replete with omega-3 fatty acids for your anti-inflammatory sojourn.

2. Fiery Shrimp and Zucchini Skewers:

Skewers showcasing boldly grilled shrimp and zucchini, delivering a delightful interplay of spice and verdant freshness to enliven your anti-inflammatory repasts.

3. Teriyaki-Glazed Haddock with Broccoli:

Haddock fillets glazed in a savory teriyaki elixir, partnered with roasted broccoli, presenting an umami-drenched and anti-inflammatory banquet.

4. Tuna and Cannellini Bean Salad:

A revitalizing salad melding delicate tuna, cannellini beans, cherry tomatoes, and a zesty lemon-herb dressing, producing a protein-laden and anti-inflammatory gastronomic marvel.

5. Creole-Seasoned Catfish with Mango Salsa:

Catfish fillets seasoned with the boldness of Creole spices, accompanied by a lively mango salsa, delivering a profusion of flavors pirouetting on your taste buds while supporting anti-inflammatory aspirations.

6. Buttery Garlic Shrimp Stir-Fry:

Shrimp waltzing in a stir-fry symphony, steeped in the luxurious embrace of garlic butter, harmonized with a kaleidoscope of vegetables, constructing a swift, delectable, and anti-inflammatory stir-fry option.

7. Zesty Cilantro-Lime Grilled Swordfish:

Swordfish steaks marinating in the zestful fusion of cilantro and lime, expertly grilled to perfection, presenting a revitalizing and anti-inflammatory aquatic jubilation.

8. Pan-Seared Diver Scallops with Asparagus:

Diver scallops meticulously seared, gracing the plate alongside tender asparagus, manifesting an opulent and anti-inflammatory culinary opus that marries flavor and nourishment.

These sumptuous seafood masterpieces are architected to elevate your anti-inflammatory epicurean odyssey. Plunge into the abyss of flavors, embrace the healthful bounty, and let these seafood wonders be a gratifying augmentation to your expedition toward holistic well-being.

★ SECTION 4: POULTRY RECIPES

Poultry-Based Recipes for Protein

Welcome to the fourth installment of the ***Anti-Inflammatory Cookbook for Beginners***, where we unfold an array of poultry-based recipes. These dishes are thoughtfully designed not only to tantalize your taste buds but also to seamlessly align with your anti-inflammatory dietary endeavors. Let's explore the world of poultry and its contribution to a flavorful and health-conscious culinary journey.

★ POULTRY RECIPES:

1. Citrus-Glazed Roast Chicken:

Roast chicken coated in a citrusy glaze, creating a succulent dish that balances robust flavors with anti-inflammatory benefits.

2. Herb-Roasted Turkey Breast:

Turkey breast delicately roasted with a medley of herbs, offering a lean and aromatic protein source for your anti-inflammatory repertoire.

3. Lemon-Honey Grilled Chicken Thighs:

Grilled chicken thighs marinated in a blend of zesty lemon and soothing honey, producing a dish that's both flavorful and anti-inflammatory.

4. Mediterranean Chicken Skewers:

Skewers laden with Mediterranean-inspired seasoned chicken, providing a savory and protein-packed anti-inflammatory feast.

5. Curry-Spiced Chicken Drumsticks:

Chicken drumsticks seasoned with an array of aromatic curry spices, delivering a bold and anti-inflammatory twist to your poultry indulgence.

6. Garlic-Herb Baked Quail:

Quail baked to perfection with a fusion of garlic and herbs, offering a sophisticated and anti-inflammatory poultry experience.

7. Sesame Ginger Turkey Burgers:

Turkey burgers infused with the nuttiness of sesame and the zing of ginger, creating a delightful and anti-inflammatory twist on a classic.

8. Balsamic Rosemary Grilled Duck Breast:

Duck breast marinated in balsamic and rosemary, grilled to perfection, presenting a rich and anti-inflammatory option for poultry enthusiasts.

Dive into the realm of poultry protein with these delectable recipes, designed to elevate your anti-inflammatory culinary escapade. Embrace the savory diversity, relish the healthful advantages, and let these poultry delights be a delightful contribution to your journey towards well-being.

★ SECTION 5: SIDE DISH RECIPES

Accompaniments for Your Meals

Welcome to the fifth section of the *Anti-Inflammatory Cookbook for Beginners*, where we explore an array of side dish recipes that complement and enhance your culinary experience. These thoughtfully crafted accompaniments are not only flavorsome but also seamlessly align with your anti-inflammatory dietary journey. Let's delve into the world of side dishes that elevate your meals to a new level.

★ SIDE DISH MARVELS:

1. Turmeric Infused Cauliflower Rice:

Cauliflower rice infused with the golden goodness of turmeric, creating a flavorful and anti-inflammatory alternative to traditional rice.

2. Garlicky Sautéed Spinach with Pine Nuts:

Spinach sautéed to perfection with garlic and adorned with pine nuts, offering a nutrient-packed and anti-inflammatory side dish.

3. Quinoa and Black Bean Stuffed Peppers:

Colorful bell peppers stuffed with a hearty mix of quinoa and black beans, providing a satisfying and anti-inflammatory accompaniment.

4. Roasted Sweet Potatoes with Cinnamon:

Sweet potatoes roasted to caramelized perfection with a sprinkle of cinnamon, presenting a delightful and anti-inflammatory twist on a classic side.

5. Mushroom and Thyme Quinoa Pilaf:

Quinoa pilaf infused with the earthy flavors of mushrooms and thyme, creating a savory and anti-inflammatory addition to your meals.

6. Asparagus and Tomato Salad with Basil Vinaigrette:

A refreshing salad featuring crisp asparagus and juicy tomatoes, dressed in a basil-infused vinaigrette, providing a burst of freshness and anti-inflammatory goodness.

7. Garlic Lemon Broccoli Florets:

Broccoli florets steamed to perfection, tossed in a zesty blend of garlic and lemon, offering a vibrant and anti-inflammatory side dish.

8. Cucumber Avocado Salsa:

A vibrant salsa combining cool cucumber and creamy avocado, offering a refreshing and anti-inflammatory topping for various dishes.

These side dish recipes are designed to enhance your anti-inflammatory meals with a burst of flavors and healthful ingredients. Explore the variety, savor the wholesome benefits, and let these accompaniments be a delightful addition to your journey toward well-being.

★ SECTION 6: SOUP RECIPES

Comforting and Nutrient-Rich Soups

Step into the sixth segment of the **Anti-Inflammatory Cookbook for Beginners,** where we explore an anthology of comforting and nutrient-dense soup recipes. These bowls of wholesome goodness are meticulously crafted not only to provide solace to your palate but also to seamlessly align with your anti-inflammatory culinary expedition. Let's immerse ourselves in the realm of soups that offer both comfort and nourishment to grace your dining table.

★ CULINARY ARTISTRY IN SOUPS:

1. Hearty Lentil and Vegetable Soup:

An assertive soup teeming with lentils, an assortment of vegetables, and a medley of aromatic spices, presenting a robust and anti-inflammatory bowl.

2. Turmeric-Infused Chicken and Rice Soup:

- Chicken and rice harmoniously blend with the golden essence of turmeric, crafting a soothing and anti-inflammatory broth.

3. Velvety Broccoli and Kale Delight:

A smooth amalgamation of broccoli and kale, forming a luscious and nutrient-packed soup that aligns with your anti-inflammatory aspirations.

4. Tomato Basil Quinoa Symphony:

A charming interplay of tomatoes, basil, and quinoa, delivering a flavorful and anti-inflammatory reinterpretation of the classic tomato soup.

5. Coconut Curry Elegance in Butternut Squash Soup:

Butternut squash soup elevated with the sophistication of coconut curry, offering a lavish and anti-inflammatory fusion of flavors.

6. Aromatic Chickpea and Spinach Harmony:

A stew featuring well-seasoned chickpeas and tender spinach leaves, creating a gratifying and anti-inflammatory bowl.

7. Earthy Mushroom Barley Sonata with Thyme:

Barley soup infused with the grounded essence of mushrooms and the herbal notes of thyme, providing a hearty and anti-inflammatory option for aficionados of soup.

8. Lively Lemon Ginger Serenade in Carrot Soup:

Carrot soup enlivened with the lively duo of zesty lemon and invigorating ginger, offering a refreshing and anti-inflammatory bowl to illuminate your day.

These culinary masterpieces in soup form are meticulously designed to bring warmth and nourishment to your anti-inflammatory gastronomic odyssey. From the robust lentils to the creamy broccoli, each bowl promises a comforting and healthful experience. Simmer, savor, and let these soups orchestrate a flavorful addition to your journey toward well-being.

★ SECTION 7: VEGETARIAN RECIPES

Plant-Based Options for All

Welcome to the seventh section of the **Anti-Inflammatory Cookbook for Beginners**, where we immerse ourselves in a collection of delightful vegetarian recipes. These plant-powered creations are not only crafted to satisfy your palate but also seamlessly align with your anti-inflammatory culinary journey. Let's embark on a culinary adventure where the vibrant world of vegetables takes center stage.

★ VEGETARIAN RECIPES:

1. Mediterranean Quinoa Salad:

A refreshing salad bursting with quinoa, cherry tomatoes, cucumber, and feta cheese, creating a symphony of flavors that complements your anti-inflammatory goals.

2. Spinach and Mushroom Stuffed Bell Peppers:

Bell peppers generously stuffed with a savory blend of spinach, mushrooms, and aromatic spices, providing a hearty and anti-inflammatory delight.

3. Chickpea and Vegetable Stir-Fry:

A colorful stir-fry featuring protein-packed chickpeas, a medley of vegetables, and a delectable array of spices, offering a quick and anti-inflammatory option.

4. Eggplant and Tomato Ratatouille:

A classic French dish celebrating the harmony of eggplant, tomatoes, zucchini, and bell peppers, delivering a flavorful and anti-inflammatory experience.

5. Creamy Avocado and Black Bean Wrap:

A satisfying wrap filled with creamy avocado, black beans, crisp vegetables, and a drizzle of lime dressing, creating a mouthwatering and anti-inflammatory ensemble.

6. Zucchini Noodles with Pesto Sauce:

Zucchini noodles coated in a vibrant pesto sauce made with basil, pine nuts, and nutritional yeast, providing a light yet satisfying anti-inflammatory alternative.

7. Sweet Potato and Chickpea Curry:

A rich and aromatic curry featuring sweet potatoes, chickpeas, and a blend of spices, creating a comforting and anti-inflammatory dish.

8. Caprese Stuffed Portobello Mushrooms:

Portobello mushrooms generously stuffed with fresh tomatoes, mozzarella, and basil, offering a delightful and anti-inflammatory twist on the classic Caprese.

These vegetarian wonders are thoughtfully designed to elevate your anti-inflammatory culinary experience. From the Mediterranean quinoa salad to the caprese-stuffed portobello mushrooms, each dish promises a harmonious blend of flavors and nutrients. Embrace the diversity, savor the freshness, and let these vegetarian creations be a delicious addition to your journey toward well-being.

★ SECTION 8: SMOOTHIE AND TEA RECIPES

Refreshing Beverages for Anytime

Welcome to the eighth section of the **Anti-Inflammatory Cookbook for Beginners**, where we explore a collection of revitalizing smoothie and tea recipes. These delightful beverages are crafted to not only quench your thirst but also seamlessly align with your anti-inflammatory culinary journey. Let's delve into a world of sips that bring both refreshment and healthful benefits to your table.

★ BEVERAGES TO SAVOR:

1. Berry Blast Smoothie:

A vibrant smoothie bursting with a medley of berries, spinach, and a touch of almond milk, offering a refreshing and anti-inflammatory blend.

2. Turmeric Ginger Citrus Tea:

A warming tea infused with turmeric, ginger, and citrusy notes, providing a soothing and anti-inflammatory beverage for relaxation.

3. Green Goddess Detox Smoothie:

A detoxifying smoothie featuring green vegetables, cucumber, and a hint of mint, creating a revitalizing and anti-inflammatory drink.

4. Hibiscus Berry Iced Tea:

Iced tea infused with hibiscus petals and a mix of berries, delivering a flavorful and antioxidant-rich anti-inflammatory refreshment.

5. Pineapple Kale Coconut Smoothie:

A tropical smoothie blending pineapple, kale, and coconut water, offering a hydrating and anti-inflammatory sip for a burst of energy.

6. Chamomile Lavender Sleep Tea:

A calming tea blend of chamomile and lavender, providing a soothing and anti-inflammatory option for relaxation before bedtime.

7. Mango Turmeric Sunshine Smoothie:

A sunshine-infused smoothie featuring mango, turmeric, and a splash of orange juice, creating a bright and anti-inflammatory sip.

8. Matcha Mint Green Tea:

Green tea with a twist of matcha and a hint of mint, offering a refreshing and antioxidant-packed anti-inflammatory beverage.

These revitalizing smoothies and teas are carefully crafted to enhance your anti-inflammatory culinary journey. From the berry blast smoothie to the chamomile lavender sleep tea, each sip promises a delightful fusion of flavors and healthful benefits. Savor the goodness, embrace the freshness, and let these beverages be a nourishing addition to your journey toward well-being.

Anti-Inflammatory For Beginners

★ SECTION 9: DESSERT AND SNACK RECIPES

Satisfying Treats and Healthy Snacks

Welcome to the ninth section of the **Anti-Inflammatory Cookbook for Beginners**, where we revel in an array of delectable treats and nourishing snacks. These indulgences are meticulously crafted not only to please your taste buds but also to seamlessly align with your anti-inflammatory lifestyle. Let's embark on a journey through a spectrum of flavors that bring delight and healthful advantages to your dining experience.

★ DELICACIES AND SNACKS TO SAVOR:

1. Rich Chocolate Berry Bites:

Petite treasures harmonizing rich chocolate with berries abundant in antioxidants, presenting a gratifying and anti-inflammatory delicacy.

2. Chia Seed Pudding Ensemble:

A tiered ensemble showcasing chia seed pudding, ripe fruits, and a sprinkling of nuts, forming a nourishing and anti-inflammatory dessert.

135

3. Cashew Butter Plantain Cookies:

Tender and chewy cookies crafted with cashew butter and ripe plantains, delivering a charming and anti-inflammatory sweet indulgence.

4. Turmeric-Infused Coconut Energy Spheres:

Energy spheres infused with the golden hues of turmeric, coconut richness, and the crunch of nuts, offering a flavorsome and anti-inflammatory snack for a swift boost.

5. Roasted Cinnamon Apple Wedges:

Apple wedges delicately roasted with a dash of cinnamon, yielding a warm and comforting, yet anti-inflammatory, snack.

6. Mediterranean Yogurt Berry Parfait:

A revitalizing parfait featuring Mediterranean yogurt, an assortment of berries, and a drizzle of honey, offering a velvety and anti-inflammatory dessert or snack alternative.

7. Matcha Bliss Bites with Almonds:

Blissful bites merging the vibrant essence of matcha with the nuttiness of almonds, creating a nurturing and anti-inflammatory treat.

8. Decadent Avocado Cocoa Mousse:

Silky cocoa mousse crafted with luscious avocado, providing an opulent and anti-inflammatory dessert with a healthful twist.

These dessert and snack compositions are meticulously shaped to introduce a touch of sweetness and contentment to your anti-inflammatory culinary escapade. Whether you yearn for a chia seed pudding ensemble or a matcha almond bliss bite, each indulgence assures a delightful interplay of flavors and healthful merits. Immerse yourself in the richness, relish the moments, and let these delectable treats and snacks become a nurturing supplement to your journey toward well-being.

★ SECTION 10: BREAD RECIPES

Baking Ideas with a Focus on Health

Welcome to the tenth section of the **Anti-Inflammatory Cookbook for Beginners**, where we embark on a journey of artisanal bread recipes. These creations are not just about the art of baking; they also prioritize health, aligning seamlessly with your anti-inflammatory lifestyle. Let's delve into the world of wholesome bread-making that adds a touch of warmth and nutrition to your culinary repertoire.

★ BREAD CREATIONS:

1. Whole Grain Seeded Loaf:

A hearty loaf combining whole grains and an assortment of seeds, offering a nutty and fiber-rich bread that complements your anti-inflammatory goals.

2. Olive and Rosemary Focaccia:

Focaccia bread infused with the flavors of olives and rosemary, creating a savory and aromatic delight with a focus on healthful ingredients.

3. Turmeric-infused Sweet Potato Bread:

Sweet potato bread enriched with the golden tones of turmeric, providing a unique and anti-inflammatory twist to your homemade bread.

4. Quinoa and Flaxseed Rolls:

Soft rolls incorporating quinoa and flaxseeds, introducing a delightful texture and an extra dose of omega-3 fatty acids for a health-conscious choice.

5. Spelt and Walnut Sourdough:

Sourdough bread featuring spelt flour and crunchy walnuts, offering a rustic and flavorful option with the benefits of reduced gluten content.

6. Millet and Cranberry Baguettes:

Baguettes crafted with millet and cranberries, delivering a subtly sweet and crunchy profile while embracing the nutritional advantages of millet.

7. Buckwheat Banana Bread:

Banana bread with the wholesome goodness of buckwheat, providing a dense and moist loaf that's gluten-free and supportive of an anti-inflammatory lifestyle.

8. Chia and Oat Artisan Bread:

Artisan-style bread combining chia seeds and oats, creating a chewy texture and adding extra fiber to make your bread experience both wholesome and delicious.

Each bread recipe is a testament to the fusion of baking craftsmanship and a health-conscious approach. From seeded loaves to turmeric-infused creations, these breads promise not just delightful flavors but also a mindful choice for your well-being. Bake, savor, and let these artisanal breads become a nourishing and delightful addition to your anti-inflammatory culinary repertoire.

Enjoy exploring these recipes and savor the flavors of your anti-inflammatory journey.

CHAPTER 7
DETAILED RECIPE ACCOUNTS

Within this chapter, we guide you through the craftsmanship of crafting delectable anti-inflammatory dishes, offering a meticulous account of each recipe. These culinary creations extend beyond mere directives; they serve as a passage toward a healthier and more vibrant version of yourself.

7.1. STEP-BY-STEP INSTRUCTIONS FOR EACH RECIPE

We furnish you with thorough, step-by-step directives for each recipe. Regardless of whether you wield the expertise of an accomplished chef or find yourself in the nascent stages of culinary exploration, our lucid and user-friendly instructions ensure the triumph of your gastronomic expedition. From initial preparation to the final presentation, we accompany you through every facet of bringing these dishes to fruition.

★ STEP-BY-STEP INSTRUCTIONS :

1. Golden Turmeric Smoothie: A Sunrise in a Glass

- ➤ **Step 1:** Gather the ingredients – turmeric, ginger, banana, and almond milk.
- ➤ **Step 2:** Peel and chop the banana, ensuring freshness and natural sweetness.
- ➤ **Step 3:** Blend the banana, turmeric, and ginger until smooth.
- ➤ **Step 4:** Pour in the almond milk, blending to the desired consistency.
- ➤ **Step 5:** Serve in a glass and savor the golden goodness.

2. Miso-Glazed Cod with Broccoli: Mastering Umami

- ➤ **Step 1:** Preheat the oven and prepare cod fillets.
- ➤ **Step 2**: Mix miso paste, soy sauce, and honey for the glaze.
- ➤ **Step 3:** Brush the cod with the miso glaze, ensuring an even coating.
- ➤ **Step 4:** Arrange broccoli around the cod for a complete meal.
- ➤ **Step 5:** Roast until cod is flaky, and broccoli is tender. Serve and enjoy!

3. Chia Seed Pudding Parfait: Layered Elegance

➤ **Step 1:** Combine chia seeds, milk, and sweetener in a bowl.

➤ **Step 2:** Stir well and refrigerate overnight to allow pudding to set.

➤ **Step 3:** Layer chia pudding with fresh fruits and nuts.

➤ **Step 4:** Repeat for a visually appealing parfait.

➤ **Step 5:** Dive in and relish the layers of healthful indulgence.

4. Olive and Rosemary Focaccia: Baking Mediterranean Flavors

➤ **Step 1:** Mix flour, yeast, water, and olive oil in a bowl.

➤ **Step 2:** Knead the dough until elastic, then let it rise.

➤ **Step 3:** Press the dough onto a baking pan, creating dimples.

➤ **Step 4:** Arrange olives and rosemary on top.

➤ **Step 5:** Bake until golden brown; savor the Mediterranean aromas.

5. Spiced Chickpea and Spinach Stew: A Simmering Comfort

- ➢ **Step 1:** Sauté onions, garlic, and spices in a pot.
- ➢ **Step 2**: Add chickpeas, tomatoes, and vegetable broth.
- ➢ **Step 3:** Simmer until chickpeas are tender.
- ➢ **Step 4:** Stir in fresh spinach until wilted.
- ➢ **Step 5:** Ladle into bowls and enjoy a comforting bowl of wellness.

6. Turmeric Coconut Energy Balls: Energizing Bites

- ➢ **Step 1:** Combine oats, coconut, nuts, and turmeric in a food processor.
- ➢ **Step 2:** Add dates and process until sticky.
- ➢ **Step 3:** Form mixture into small balls.
- ➢ **Step 4**: Refrigerate to set and enhance flavors.
- ➢ **Step 5:** Grab a ball for a quick, energizing bite.

This comprehensive set of instructions serves not just as a manual for your hands in the culinary domain but also unveils the narratives embedded within every recipe. Immerse yourself in the intricacies, welcome the procedural intricacies, and permit the culinary craft to become an enchanting facet of your journey through the realm of anti-inflammatory gastronomy.

7.2. NUTRITIONAL INFORMATION FOR EVERY DISH

Recognizing the nutritional composition of your meals constitutes a pivotal aspect of an anti-inflammatory dietary regimen. For every recipe featured, we present an in-depth analysis of its nutritional constituents, encompassing details such as calories, macronutrients, vitamins, and minerals. This knowledge empowers you to make judicious choices and monitor your intake as you progress toward enhanced well-being.

Example: Explore the gratification of our Grilled Salmon with Lemon and Dill, where the sensory pleasure is not only derived from its flavor but also from the bestowal of essential omega-3 fatty acids, lean protein, and crucial vitamins and minerals.

7.3. COOKING TIPS AND VARIATIONS

Enhance your culinary skills with practical cooking tips and creative variations that elevate the anti-inflammatory cooking experience. For example, share insights on optimal ingredient substitutions, efficient kitchen techniques, or innovative flavor enhancements, allowing beginners to customize recipes while maintaining the healthful essence of the anti-inflammatory approach.

7.4. SERVING SUGGESTIONS AND PRESENTATION IDEAS

Elevate your anti-inflammatory creations with inspiring serving suggestions and presentation ideas. For instance, explore the art of garnishing to add a pop of color, suggest complementary side dishes that enhance the overall dining experience, or propose creative plating techniques that turn each meal into a visual masterpiece.

These enhancements will not only delight the palate but also make the anti-inflammatory culinary journey a feast for the eyes.

For our Chia Seed Pudding with Fresh Berries, we'll recommend garnishing with extra berries and a drizzle of honey to create an inviting and vibrant presentation.

Upon concluding this chapter, you'll not only possess an array of recipes but also wield a culinary toolkit that enables the creation of meals that are not merely health-conscious but also a sensory delight. Relish the entire process – from the culinary artistry to the presentation and the subsequent enjoyment of each dish – as you traverse further on your anti-inflammatory journey.

CHAPTER 8
CONCLUSION

In this ultimate chapter, we stand at the pinnacle of your exploration through the realm of anti-inflammatory eating. You've delved into the importance of this dietary approach, mastered the art of informed decision-making, and honed your skills in crafting nourishing meals. Now, let's contemplate your steadfast commitment to this lifestyle and cast our gaze forward.

8.1. NURTURING A LASTING ANTI-INFLAMMATORY LIFESTYLE

Fostering an anti-inflammatory lifestyle transcends momentary efforts; it's a sustained dedication to your health and overall well-being. Within this chapter, we provide counsel on how to perpetuate this commitment, even in the face of challenges and enticements. Offering insights on seamlessly integrating anti-inflammatory principles into your daily regimen, we aim to make it an inherent part of your routine. By comprehending the far-reaching impact on your health, you'll discover the impetus to persevere.

8.2. FUTURE HEALTH AND WELLNESS GOALS

Your expedition doesn't culminate at this juncture. In this segment, we prompt you to contemplate your future health and wellness aspirations. Anti-inflammatory eating constitutes merely one facet of a holistic well-being approach. We'll explore ways for you to establish and attain these goals, whether it involves maintaining a balanced weight, navigating stress, or enhancing your physical fitness. Your commitment to an anti-inflammatory lifestyle forms the groundwork upon which you can construct a future marked by enhanced health and contentment.

8.3. CELEBRATING YOUR SUCCESS AND MILESTONES

Commending achievements is an integral component of any odyssey. In this section, we urge you to recognize your triumphs, irrespective of their scale. Be it seamlessly incorporating anti-inflammatory meals into your weekly routine or relishing heightened energy levels and overall well-being, each milestone merits acknowledgment. We'll propose avenues for rewarding yourself and acknowledging your unwavering commitment to a healthier lifestyle.

As you draw the curtains on this book, it's not merely the conclusion of a chapter; it signifies the commencement of an enduring path towards health and vitality.

We trust that the knowledge and tools you've acquired will be steadfast companions on your journey, and that anti-inflammatory eating will seamlessly integrate into the fabric of your life. Congratulations on taking this stride toward improved health, and may the chapters that unfold in your future be adorned with triumphs, well-being, and joy.

CHAPTER 9
SUPPLEMENTARY MATERIALS

Within this comprehensive appendix, you'll uncover a multitude of supplementary resources and tools designed to strengthen your foray into anti-inflammatory practices. These provisions are meticulously created to enhance your understanding, simplify your culinary pursuits, and provide seamless access to the recipes that align with your preferences.

9.1. CULINARY LEXICON

Navigating the realm of culinary arts can often feel akin to entering uncharted territory, replete with unfamiliar expressions and methodologies. Within this segment, we've assembled a culinary lexicon to unravel the intricacies of culinary terminology. From discerning the nuances between sautéing and simmering to honing indispensable knife techniques, this lexicon stands as your culinary compendium.

9.2. SOURCE MATERIALS AND CITATIONS

This is a treasure trove of meticulously researched and cited references. It offers a comprehensive array of reputable sources, studies, and expert opinions that validate and support the nutritional information, culinary insights, and health benefits outlined in the cookbook. These meticulously curated citations serve as the backbone, providing a reliable and scientifically-backed foundation for the anti-inflammatory principles guiding your culinary journey towards improved health and well-being.

9.3. UTENSILS AND APPARATUS FOR YOUR CULINARY HAVEN

Discover the Necessary Utensils and Gear for Your Culinary Sanctuary within the pages of this **Anti-Inflammatory Cookbook for Beginners**. Reveal the core tools and equipment that aim not only to streamline your cooking expedition but also to elevate your engagement in crafting delectable and health-conscious anti-inflammatory dishes. Spanning from adaptable blades to specific culinary contraptions, this manual is crafted to assist novices in outfitting their kitchens for triumph, guaranteeing a smooth and pleasurable culinary escapade.

9.4. QUICK-REFERENCE CATALOG FOR RECIPES

This is a convenient compendium designed to streamline your culinary experience. This comprehensive catalog is your go-to resource, offering a quick and easy way to navigate through the diverse range of anti-inflammatory recipes featured in the book. With categorization by meal types, dietary preferences, and flavors, this catalog ensures swift access to a plethora of delicious and health-conscious recipes, empowering you to effortlessly plan and prepare meals that suit your taste, lifestyle, and dietary needs.

This supplementary annex is crafted to serve as your culinary compatriot, delivering the implements and materials requisite for you to persist in your anti-inflammatory expedition with assurance and simplicity. With a culinary lexicon to demystify culinary vernacular, supplementary materials to deepen your insight, suggestions for indispensable kitchen instruments, and a recipe catalog for swift retrieval, you'll possess everything essential to embrace anti-inflammatory cooking as an enduring lifestyle.

CHAPTER 10
GRATITUDE

As we reach the culmination of this expedition, we feel compelled to convey our profound gratitude to the individuals and entities whose indispensable contributions breathed life into the **"Anti-Inflammatory Cookbook for Beginners."** Their steadfast backing, unwavering commitment, and wellsprings of inspiration have been the catalysts propelling the genesis of this literary endeavor.

We wish to extend our heartfelt thanks to:

- Our families, whose steadfast support and encouragement have been a constant throughout this odyssey.

- The skilled chefs, nutritionists, and experts who graciously shared their wealth of knowledge and insights, contributing to the substance of this book.

- The industrious editorial and design teams whose relentless efforts ensured that this book is not just informative but also visually captivating.

- The numerous volunteers who selflessly served as recipe testers, providing invaluable feedback to refine the culinary masterpieces within these pages.

- Our readers and supporters, whose enthusiasm for embracing an anti-inflammatory lifestyle has been a tremendous source of inspiration, propelling us to share our passion for wholesome eating.

- The publishing and distribution partners whose collaboration has made it possible for this book to reach readers globally.

- The researchers and authors whose groundbreaking work has laid the foundation for the anti-inflammatory diet movement.

And, most importantly, to you, the reader, for embarking on this expedition toward improved health and wellness alongside us. Your curiosity, dedication, and commitment to enhancing your well-being are the driving forces behind this book.

This book is dedicated to each and every one of you. May it serve as a compass and wellspring of inspiration as you navigate toward a healthier and more vibrant life.

Thank you for being an integral part of this journey, and we eagerly anticipate continuing to support your health and wellness aspirations.

THE END

www.ingramcontent.com/pod-product-compliance
Lightning Source LLC
Chambersburg PA
CBHW072207290526
45794CB00004B/1688